PRAISE FOR *STRETCHING YOUR WAY TO A PAIN-FREE LIFE*

"Aaron brought the freedom of pain-free movement to my family for over ten years with his specialized stretches. Now he's sharing his unique stretching program to help everyone enjoy more fluid movement. I highly recommend *Stretching Your Way to a Pain-Free Life* to anyone wanting to maintain an active and healthy lifestyle."

—Lonnie Ali
Wife of Muhammad Ali

"As we age, we get less flexible, and our bodies become stiffer, tighter, and slower moving. Aaron Taylor, a 20-year veteran flexibility coach, brilliantly shares how to stretch your way to less pain, greater flexibility and mobility, and new levels of free movement. To keep mobile, flexible, and bodily free, read this book."

—Mark Victor Hansen
World's bestselling author with 500,000,000 books sold;
best known for co-creating the *Chicken Soup for the Soul* series

"Aaron has worked with my aches and pains for nearly 20 years. I LOVE how he provides information in this book that we can all understand and relate to. He has continued to help me, and I know *Stretching Your Way to a Pain-Free Life* will help you as well!"

—Betsy King
LPGA Hall of Fame Member
2007 Solheim Cup Captain

"As professional golfers, we understand how important mobility and flexibility are. Aaron takes you through simple and effective stretching techniques that will allow your body to move more freely and feel younger."

—Arron & Angie Oberholser
Retired PGA Tour and LPGA Tour

"What Aaron Taylor has presented here is a comprehensive, easy-to-understand guide to all types of stretching. He not only shows us how to stretch properly, but simply explains the importance of stretching to maximize performance and well-being. This book can help everyone from the weekend warrior to the professional athlete like myself."

—Erik Hanson
Former MLB pitcher; competitive amateur golfer

STRETCHING YOUR WAY TO A PAIN-FREE LIFE

ILLUSTRATED STRETCHES
for Sports, Medical Conditions and Specific Muscle Groups

AARON TAYLOR

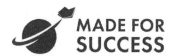

MADE FOR
SUCCESS

Made for Success Publishing
P.O. Box 1775 Issaquah, WA 98027
www.MadeForSuccessPublishing.com

Distributed by Made for Success Publishing

First Printing

Library of Congress Cataloging-in-Publication data

Taylor, Aaron

Stretching Your Way to a Pain-Free Life:
Illustrated Stretches for Sports, Medical Conditions and Specific Muscle Groups
p. cm.

LCCN: 2021938425

ISBN: 978-1-64146-585-4 (*Paperback*)
ISBN: 978-1-64146-586-1 (*ebook*)

Printed in the United States of America

For further information contact Made for Success Publishing
+14255266480 or email service@madeforsuccess.net

TABLE OF CONTENTS

Acknowledgements

I have had a few people that have been very instrumental in my life, none more so than my entire family. Thank you for your constant support and encouragement. My mom and dad are both retired teachers and I am sure they did not know their son would write a book! Surprise! This book is to both of you. Thank you for all you have provided me throughout my entire life, I could not have asked for better parents.

To my wonderful wife Stephanie and the best sons in the world, Peyton and Gavin. Thank you for being you. You were all so patient with me throughout this entire process, always encouraging me to keep going and listening to my constant complaints about the computer and my lack of knowledge of how to use it. Because of all your help, I am better now though, right?

An incredibly special thank you to everyone who assisted me with this book. To all my models, Betsy King, Erik Hanson, Laney, Dan, Derek, and Kristin, thank you for all your time taking pictures. I hope your bodies felt better after all that stretching. To Mary for all your hard work editing my book for the first time. I know you did me a great favor and I will never forget it! To Deedee Heathman and everyone at Made For Success Publishing, THANK YOU! It was an absolute pleasure working you all. The book turned out amazing.

Last but definitely not least, to all of my clients that badgered me to get this book done, thank you. It has been a pleasure working with you all these past 20 years. Without you, this book would not have been written. A special thank you to Harvey Mackay who has been on me for nearly 20 years to write a book. Here it is Harvey, sorry it took a while, but it is done...Finally! You and Carol Ann have a special place in my life. Thank you for everything!

INTRODUCTION

There's no magic trick to reverse aging, but there *is* a technique so effective that it can make you feel like you've just taken years off your age. Or, more specifically, in the case of my 85-year old client, taken 60 years off your age! That's exactly what happened after my client was introduced to a stretching program for the first time in his life. He completed his first series of stretches, looked at me incredulously, and said, "I feel like I am in my 20s again!"

Now, that's not going to be everyone's experience, and I realize that stretching isn't a cure-all, but a proper stretching program, executed correctly, can be life-changing. I've worked with all kinds of people over my 20-year career, and my favorite words to hear are, "I don't hurt anymore!" With a regular stretching program, you, too, can eliminate or greatly reduce pain.

I have been around the athletic scene my entire life. From the age of 5, I remember going to football practice with my dad, who was the coach, where I would catch crawdads in a little stream by the field and occasionally watch those great, big high school football players practice. As I grew older, my mom and dad provided me with the opportunity to participate in football, basketball, wrestling, baseball, soccer, and golf. Wow, good luck doing all of that now! Obviously, I had to make some choices and decide which one of those sports I was going to continue. Although I loved all of them, I played basketball to stay in shape and get through the cold winters in Alamosa, Colorado, and golf where I knew my future lay. I played golf all through high school and college. As I look back on those wonderful years, and knowing what I know now, I realize we spent very little time in one of the most important physical aspects, not only in sports, but in life: stretching.

After my college career was over, I moved to drier pastures down in Scottsdale, Arizona. I became a flexibility specialist and had the opportunity to work with some of the greatest names in sport and entertainment history. As you can imagine,

Alamosa, Colorado didn't have many famous people living there (more like *zero*), so I had to try very hard not to be completely in awe of these people while working with them. I worked for 8-12 hours a day, stretching people, learning how the human body moves, and more importantly, learning about all the issues people deal with on a daily basis due to a lack of mobility. I have been able to work with all types, from professional athletes to couch potatoes, ages 12 years old to 90 years young, and weekend warriors to individuals afflicted with Parkinson's disease or joint replacements. However, the greatest thing of all through my near 20 years of work is that I have witnessed time and time again the benefits of a regular stretching program.

Although stretching has become more prevalent, people still don't have a good handle on how to stretch. My goal with this book is to continue what I have been able to do in the last 20 years, and that is to help people from all walks of life feel and move better. No matter your age or athletic ability, this book will give you the basic knowledge of how stretching works, the benefits of stretching, different types of stretching techniques, and even specific foods you can eat that can help you attain your goals. The hundreds of stretches that this book contains will give you many choices so that you never get bored and give up on improving your wellbeing. Toward the end of this book, I have provided my favorite daily stretching routines, stretching routines that can assist you with specific ailments, and sport-specific routines.

I truly hope that with the assistance of this book, you will make stretching a daily habit.

FOREWORD

I had the pleasure of meeting Aaron almost 20 years ago. I was talking with a wonderful friend of mine from the Twin Cities who happens to be one of the best female golfers to ever come out of the state of Minnesota. Through conversation, she asked me if I had ever been stretched. She then lay huge praise on Aaron and told me I had to give him a call.

I have always been active. I have run ten marathons, played competitive tennis and collegiate golf. Like all golfers, I am always looking for any advantage, including those elusive ten extra yards. Stretching sounded great to me, so I called the very next day.

During our first visit, I assumed that his "routine" would be like all other stretching routines, maybe geared a bit more towards golf. He walks in carrying a portable massage table and asks me to lay on my back. Our one-hour session flew by. The way I felt after my time with Aaron was such a dramatic change that I knew this routine would become part of my everyday life. It was that good!

Aaron's new book, *Stretching Your Way to a Pain-Free Life*, really explains and teaches exactly what he did for me! He has taken his year of experience working with some of the biggest names in sports and entertainment, including Muhammad Ali, for 12 years and shared the "How-To's" of stretching with accompanying illustrations. He is very well respected in the industry and has appeared in *American Fitness magazine* and *Sports Illustrated*.

I am excited about Aaron's book for a couple of reasons; First, I have been working with Aaron for over 20 years. He has become a bit of a fixture in the Mackay household and second because the way he teaches stretching is unique and life-changing. Think of being able to do things you haven't been able to for years, just by stretching, or upping your game, whatever it may be, by learning his stretches.

He provides stretches explicitly designed for sports and stretches broken up by the parts of the body. The book is straightforward to read, and the stretches are easy to follow.

Whenever I speak to anyone having any flexibility issues, I send them his way. If you don't get the privilege of working with Aaron directly, his book is the next best thing.

Harvey Mackay

BENEFITS OF STRETCHING

In recent years, many people have discovered the benefits of stretching through techniques like yoga and Pilates. But stretching has had a long history of benefiting athletes by helping them reach their optimum performance. For years, we've witnessed athletes getting stretched by a coach or a trainer before an important sporting event. While it might escape you at first glance, there is a profound advantage to stretching and improving your overall body movement. I like to think that better movement is the building block to complete fitness and an individual's overall wellbeing—no matter your age or athletic ability. By staying consistent with a stretching program, you can benefit in the following ways:

Better Range of Motion: Range of motion refers to the amount of movement we have in our joints. As a muscle shortens and becomes stiff, it creates tension not just in the muscle, but also in the tendons and ligaments. As our connective tissues tighten, they place more tension on our joints, which can cause less range of motion as well as additional friction and rubbing within the joint.

Better Blood and Oxygen Circulation: Vasoconstriction is a term used to describe the narrowing of a blood vessel due to the tightening of the surrounding muscle).[1] When a person stretches properly and allows the muscle to relax, the muscle can release the proverbial chokehold it has on the blood vessels, allowing for better circulation of blood and oxygen. Poor circulation can cause pain and cramp in your muscles, as well as tingling in your hands and feet. As our red blood cells collect the oxygen, it is carried off throughout our body to our body's tissue. Oxygen can then help to counteract the buildup of lactic acid in the muscle, which can lead to faster recovery.

Less Arthritic Pain: Arthritis is inflammation of your joints, which causes stiffness and pain. When a joint becomes stiff, it creates more friction on your cartilage, ultimately causing it to break down. In severe cases, it breaks down the cartilage completely, causing bone-on-bone rubbing in your joint. Due to the pain, people tend to limit their movement, which creates tighter muscles, and produces more tension and pain in the joint. Instead, we should focus on some light, easy stretches, so your muscles can relax enough to take some of that tension off your joints.

Reduced Stress and Anxiety: We are living in a fast-paced world, constantly working, trying to get ahead, and taking care of the needs of our loved ones, all of which can be a recipe for building stress and anxiety. Stress and anxiety can raise your heart rate and produce tension in the muscles, which creates tightness. Taking 20-30 minutes off per day to stretch and focus on your needs allows you to slow down, breathe, and relax. As your heart rate lowers and you increase your circulation, you can relieve the tension in your muscles.

Fewer Aches and Pains: One of the biggest causes of all of our little aches and pains is being sedentary. We sit at work at our desks all day (which tightens the muscles in our body), and then we go home and rest our aches and pains again by sitting or lying down on the couch. Our body was made to move! Stretching can take away most of the pressure that has been placed on our muscles, joints, tendons, and ligaments from sitting and allows our body to move more freely.

Improved Posture: I would like to share a little story about this benefit. For as long as I have been working with individuals on their stretching and body movement, my clients have had a common question.

"Will I get taller?"

After hearing this question nearly every week, I started to think that it was a possibility, so I began measuring everybody before and after I stretched them. Funny enough, I found that 100% of my clients were indeed taller after I worked with them. Of course, just like anything else, they didn't believe me. So, I decided that I was going to prove it to them by taking a picture of them before and after I stretched them standing in front of a postural analysis grid chart. Now I had visual proof of them growing in some cases an inch in only a 30- or 60-minute session.

Now, obviously, we aren't elongating the skeletal structure of the human body and making them taller by stretching. As our muscles get tighter, our body wants to pull down and forward, causing our shoulders to round forward and our body to sink toward the ground. What we are doing through stretching is elongating all those muscles that place pressure on all of our joints, which, again, causes less spacing in our joints and creates friction. In essence, we are allowing more room in the joint, which elongates and straightens our body.

The pictures below show an individual before and after successively getting stretched. Also, make sure to notice that the cane is in the picture before getting stretched, but not in the picture after getting stretched!

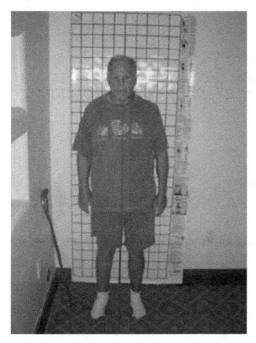 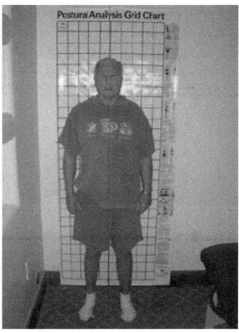

Better Mental Focus: As we stretch, or do any kind of exercise, for that matter, our brain releases endorphins. Produced in the pituitary gland and the hypothalamus, endorphins are the body's natural feel-good chemical. It can help to alleviate pain, lessen depression, and boost your mental focus.

Less Sciatic Pain: The sciatic nerve is the longest nerve in the human body, starting in the lower back and extending all the way down into the foot. Though many problems can be associated with pressure on the nerve in the lower back, which may be caused by a disc problem, sciatic issues can also be associated with tension within the muscles. Stretching the muscles within the buttocks, primarily the piriformis, which overlaps the sciatic nerve, can help to alleviate sciatic nerve pain.

Reduced Chance of Injury and Enhanced Performance: I wanted to put these two together because I believe they work hand in hand. I think that we can all agree that a flexible body moves more freely and has fewer restrictions. Whether you are just trying to get up out of your chair, squatting down to pick up a dumbbell, or trying to hit a 300-yard drive, your flexibility plays a key role in how well these tasks are executed.

As we have discussed previously, the tighter our muscles are, the less range of motion we have in our bodies. Watch people as they walk, get out of a chair, or bend over to pick something up off the ground. If you watch closely, you will start to see people walking bent over at the waist or with their feet pointed out; you will see people using anything they can to help themselves out of a chair, and you will see all kinds of ways people try to get down toward the floor.

FACTORS AFFECTING FLEXIBILITY

Over the course of my career, I have learned that we are not created equal physically. Some people can stretch every day of their life and not have as much flexibility as someone who seldom stretches. As we get older, we start to see and feel changes within our body and how it works, or worse yet, how it doesn't work! The following factors can give us some insight into these differences.

Age: The importance of staying active and stretching becomes greater as we get older. As we age, our muscles tend to thicken and become more fibrous, making it more difficult for us to move freely. As our metabolism slows, our muscles begin to atrophy as we become less active and start to gain weight. Sarcopenia is a term used to describe the loss of skeletal muscle due to age. According to Crowther, "As the body ages, muscle bulk and strength decline slowly, beginning as early as age 50, with loss of about 1% per year thereafter."[2] On top of it all, we tend to change the way we eat, and we also start drinking less water. This is all a recipe for disaster for not only our flexibility, but how our body feels in general.

Gender: Sorry men, women tend to be more flexible than we are. Men typically have more muscle mass than women. Women also have a shallower pelvis, which in turn allows for better movement in the hips. On top of this, women produce hormones (i.e., estrogen) that tend to loosen connective tissue in the body.

Connective Tissue: We have two primary types of connective tissue that can negatively or positively affect an individuals' movement and flexibility. The first of these is collagenous tissue, which is composed primarily of fibrous proteins called collagen. Found primarily in the tendons, ligaments, and skin, collagenous tissue helps to provide strength and support in our body. However, it is not very flexible, and that can limit our range of motion.

The other type of connective tissue is elastic tissue, which is composed primarily of a different kind of protein fiber called elastin. The amount of elastic tissue is really what determines our range of motion. The more we have, the more we can move.

Genetics: We see it every day we watch professional sports. Athletes at the highest level were born physically gifted. Don't get me wrong, they also worked very hard to get to that level, but how is it that a 6'5" man who weighs 350 pounds can be so strong, do splits, and touch his chest on the floor (I have seen it)? When we are born, our connective tissue (i.e., muscles, tendons, and ligaments) can not only differ in elasticity but also in length. These differences can cause a person's tightness.

Joint Structure: As we have discussed previously, an individuals' flexibility and range of motion are directly related to the joints and the connective tissue surrounding them. We have three different classifications of joints:

- **Synovial Joints:** The most common joint in the body, including the knee, hip, wrist, elbow, and shoulder. Each synovial joint is surrounded by a capsule that seals and provides lubrication and stability to the joint. These joints also have more range of motion than our other joints.
- **Cartilaginous Joints:** This joint binds bones together through bands of cartilage, providing a limited range of motion. The intervertebral discs of the spine and the sternocostal joint in the ribs are two examples[3]
- **Fibrous Joints:** Having no joint cavity, fibrous joints are connected by fibrous connective tissue and have no movement. An example of a fibrous joint would be the sutures of the skull bones.

Injuries: Every year as a sports fan, you hear about it, pulled hamstrings, torn pectoral muscles, injuries to the shoulders and back, and the list goes on. As sports fans, we get upset when our favorite players get hurt and can't play, and many times, we get even more upset when they don't come back when we think they should. We need to remember that any time we have an injury, not only do we need to allow it to heal, but then we need to rehab the injury. Whether it is in the muscle, joint, or bone, we start to develop scar tissue. Scar tissue is a more dense and fibrous tissue that protects the injury but doesn't allow it to move very freely. Injuries to a muscle, or any other connective tissue, can result in fibrosis (the development of scar tissue or thickening of the tissue to heal). On the positive side, the injured area is healed and feels better, but on the negative side, it also feels tighter and doesn't move as easily.

Diet: At this point in our lives, we should all understand that eating right and putting healthy food in our bodies is essential for our overall wellbeing. Eating healthy foods helps to cleanse our bodies of waste that can become toxic. In this section, I just want to touch briefly on several items that can truly help us gain more benefits in our stretching program.

Vitamin D: Vitamin D is essential for the absorption of calcium. Without the appropriate levels of this vitamin, only 10-15% of calcium and 60% of phosphorus can be absorbed. A vitamin D deficiency can precipitate a decrease in bone mineral density (osteopenia), softening of the bones (osteomalacia), decrease in bone strength (osteoporosis), as well as muscle weakness, which can cause more falls, greatly increasing the risk of fractures and other injuries.

We can get a considerable amount of vitamin D from the sun; however, using sunscreen reduces its absorption into the body by as much as 99%.[4] This is why we truly need to have a plan for what we eat daily. Foods that are higher in vitamin D are:

Salmon   Portobellos   Almondmilk   Tofu

**Food lists taken from My Food Data.

Vitamin C: Vitamin C is essential in the formation and maintenance of collagen. Collagen is the primary structural protein that is needed for the growth and repair of bone, skin, and connective tissue (tendons, ligaments, muscles, blood vessels). A vitamin C deficiency can slow your metabolism, making your body more fatigued.

Found in fruits and vegetables, vitamin C is best eaten in its raw form as cooking destroys most of the vitamins.[5] Foods high in vitamin C are:

Peppers   Kale   Mango   Oranges

Vitamin B: B vitamins contribute to the metabolism of protein and are also responsible for the production of energy in our body. A lack of specific B vitamins such as B1, B5, and B6 can also lead to an individual having muscle cramps. Vitamin B12, on the other hand, helps in the development of red blood cells (red blood cells carry oxygen throughout our body). Foods high in vitamin B are:

Tuna   Milk   Eggs   Beef

Vitamin E: Vitamin E assists in the formation of red blood cells and is also necessary for the maintenance of skeletal, cardiac, and smooth muscle. Individuals with poor eating habits who tend to eat large amounts of processed foods, sugar, and alcohol tend to develop deficiencies, which can lead to fatigue. Foods that are high in vitamin E are:

| Olive Oil | Peanut Butter | Avocados | Legumes |

Calcium: Calcium assists in maintaining bone strength, blood clotting, nerve impulses (our reaction or movement that is caused by an outside stimulus causes a muscle to contract), as well as PH and blood pressure control. A lack of calcium can result in fractures and osteoporosis. A few foods higher in calcium are:

| Milk Products | Broccoli | Clams | Oatmeal |

Iron: Iron plays a critical role in carrying oxygen to cells and removing carbon dioxide. A deficiency will cause a person to feel fatigued, thus inhibiting their exercise potential. Tea, coffee, and chocolate can inhibit iron absorption. Foods high in iron are:

| Liver | Red Meat | Nuts | Spinach |

Potassium: Potassium regulates water balance in the body, helps to generate muscle contractions, and regulates the heartbeat. A lack of potassium can cause fatigue, muscle weakness, and slower reflexes. Foods higher in potassium are:

| Bananas | Sweet Potatoes | Peaches | Oranges |

Sodium: Sodium is an electrolyte that assists in facilitating muscle contraction and nerve impulses and is also closely tied with the movement and balance of water throughout the body. Due to the abundance of sodium in practically all of the food we eat, we typically don't have sodium deficiencies. That being said, if you do have a deficiency, your symptoms could include cramps, nausea, and dizziness. A few healthy sources of sodium are:

| Beets | Cantaloupe | Shrimp | Spinach |

The RDA for sodium is 2,300 mg per day, and only 1500 mg for those with high blood pressure.[6]

Magnesium: Magnesium, another key mineral found within the body, plays a critical role in bone development and energy production. Levels of magnesium can be negatively affected by increased consumption of coffee, tea, soda, as well as alcohol. Refined sugar from sweets and desserts can cause magnesium to even be excreted from the body. Symptoms of a deficiency can include cramps, chronic pain, poor sleep, inflammation, and even depression. The RDA of magnesium is 400 mg for adults. Try eating these foods that are rich in magnesium:

Almonds   Black Beans   Brown Rice   Quinoa

Water: It is said that the human body is approximately 60% water, so why don't we drink enough even though we all know it is essential for life? I want you to ask yourself: *Am I drinking enough water?* I always tell my clients if you have to think about it, chances are you aren't getting enough.

Not only does water transport nutrients and minerals throughout the body, but it also helps to regulate body temperature, lubricate our joints, and assist our vital organs in performing more efficiently. Just a 2% decrease of water in our body can cause fatigue, loss of coordination, decreased mental focus, irritability, dry skin, elevated body temperature, cramps, loss of strength and endurance, and can cause our body to become toxic, which makes it difficult for our body to move and perform correctly.

So how important is water for your muscles and other connective tissues? I think a great analogy is a piece of beef jerky. Strange, I know, but what is beef jerky? It is dehydrated meat or tissue—it doesn't have any water in it, so it is firm, not very flexible, and tears pretty easily. Now compare that to a raw steak!

Sugar: Sugar is perhaps the best-tasting, most dangerous substance we have access to. In fact, many of us have a love/hate relationship with it. It is unfortunate that something that can taste so good can be so harmful! You may have heard this before, but sugar is sometimes referred to as an "empty calorie," which means that it doesn't contain any nutritional value such as proteins, minerals, or vitamins.

According to the USDA, the average American consumes roughly 47 pounds of cane sugar and 35 pounds of high fructose corn syrup per year. YIKES! I know, I know, your brain is telling you that you want it. However, if this is the case, then you need to be aware of what is going on in the brain. Dopamine and serotonin are two chemicals that are produced in the brain that can be contributing factors to sugar addiction. Sugar can trigger the production of dopamine while decreases in serotonin can cause sugar cravings. Please remember that the more you feed your cravings, the more you want it! Braverman mentions that "Serotonin is made from tryptophan, and tryptophan supplementation frequently decreases sugar craving,"[7] so if you are suffering from too much sugar, you may want to look at those foods again that are high in tryptophan.

So how does sugar affect our body? As we eat it, the sugar enters into our bloodstream, making our body more acidic. Calcium and magnesium can be leached from our bones and muscles, causing even weaker bones, muscle cramps, muscle tension, and, ultimately, muscle tightness. It can also cause an insulin spike, which can lead to inflammation throughout our body. Some of the more serious side effects of a sugar-rich diet can be Type 2 diabetes, obesity, depression, hypertension, and heart disease. According to the American Heart Association, they recommend that women have 6 tsp, while men have 9 tsp. per day. Here is a list that may shock you, according to an article entitled, "18 Foods and Drinks That Are Surprisingly High In Sugar":[8]

- Bottled smoothies (can contain 96 grams of sugar)
- Yogurt
- Condiments, i.e., Ketchup and BBQ sauce
- Energy drinks
- Protein bars

Amount of Exercise: This is very simple. If you don't use it, you lose it. Typically, active people tend to be more flexible and move better than those who are sedentary. As we discussed earlier, active people tend to have better oxygen and blood flow throughout the body. This, along with their body's connective tissue being in better shape, allows for better movement and flexibility.

Body Temperature: I prefer my clients to come ready to stretch. This means their body is already warmed up. Take 5-10 minutes on the treadmill, bike, or even in a hot shower to get ready to stretch.

Improper Breathing: Isn't it funny how something that comes so naturally to us is one of the most misused aspects of fitness and therapy? We see it all the time in the gym and on our therapy tables: people not breathing correctly, or even holding their breath. Believe it or not, this only tightens your muscles! When we breathe properly, our oxygen levels increase, which allows our red blood cells to collect and carry it throughout our body to our body's tissue. Proper breathing can also help to:

- Boost energy levels
- Improve stamina
- Counteract acids (e.g., lactic acid)
- Release toxins
- Relieve tension
- Relax the mind
- Relieve stress and anxiety
- Loosen muscles
- Relieve pain
- Increase muscle strength and flexibility
- Strengthen your immune system
- Metabolize vitamins and nutrients (leads to faster recovery)
- Increase blood flow
- Increase athletic ability
- Reduce tissue swelling

Physical Diagnosis: Unfortunately, we won't live a life without some sort of physical ailment. We can deal with the occasional strain and sprain, but the life of many people changes drastically after they are diagnosed with something unexpected. Parkinson's disease, Guillain-Barre syndrome, and stiff-person syndrome are just a few movement disorders with which we can be diagnosed. All of these disorders will affect how a person moves and the flexibility of the connective tissue in the body.

Sleep: Perhaps one of the most overlooked aspects of our physical health is sleep. We are all trying to get ahead in life, so we just continue to pile up more and more activities. As our list of activities continues to grow, and we can't find more time in the day to accomplish everything we set out for, we have no alternative other than to steal those precious hours at night. The lack of sleep affects us mentally and emotionally, and it also plays a necessary role in our physical health. Sleep, and in particular, *deep sleep*, not only helps to boost muscle growth and repair, but it promotes healing and repair of the heart and blood vessels as well.[9]

According to the National Sleep Foundation, children need approximately 9-11 hours of sleep, teens between the ages of 14-17 need 8-10 hours, adults should get between 7-9 hours, and individuals who are 65 and older should have at least 7-8 hours of sleep.

What we consume in our daily diet can affect our sleeping habits as well. Try to lessen your intake or avoid eating and drinking the biggest offenders, such as sugar and caffeine. Instead, try eating foods that are rich in vitamin D, magnesium, and calcium, as they can assist in relaxing the body. Another item you may want to introduce into your diet is tryptophan. Tryptophan is an amino acid that is used in the synthesis of serotonin and melatonin, both of which are thought to be involved in the regulation of sleep. Foods that are high in tryptophan are:

Turkey   Chicken   Bananas   Eggs

STRETCHING METHODS

Stretching has many different methods from which you can choose. Although they all have a place in an individual's fitness plan, they may not be for everyone. The methods I highly recommend are static and passive stretching. They are the most common forms of stretching and tend to be a little safer and more relaxing. My personal favorite forms of stretching are dynamic and PNF. I believe everyone can benefit from these two methods, but people have a tendency to think that only athletes do them, so they stay away. I, however, strongly urge you to try them. The last method of stretching is ballistic. I don't cover this much because in all honesty, I am not a big fan. The following is a list of the forms of stretching I'll be teaching you throughout this book.

Static Stretching: Static stretching is a method of stretching your muscles at rest, and is composed of various techniques that allow you to take a muscle to its optimal length and hold the position for 20-30 seconds. This method of stretching is what people typically perform and is a wonderful way to stretch out and relax after a workout. Some advantages of this method include:

- Safest form of stretching
- Enables you to sink into your stretch and focus on the area being stretched
- Allows for better mind and body relaxation
- Can create a permanent change in the length of the muscle
- Allows the person to focus more on proper breathing
- If done correctly, the stretch reflex does not initiate
- Can create a GTO (Golgi tendon organ – a sensory organ that senses changes in muscle tension) response

Passive Stretching: Similar to static stretching, passive stretching allows your body to relax fully during your stretch while you hold the position for 20-30 seconds. The difference between the two methods is that passive stretching utilizes an outside force to assist you with the stretch, such as:

- A partner
- Straps and towels
- Your hands, feet, and legs
- Body weight

Ballistic Stretching: Ballistic stretching uses bouncing-type movements to stretch the muscle, and the end position is not held. Using the standing toe touch as an example, when you bend forward at the hips to touch your toes instead of holding the position, you bounce down toward your feet and then right back up again. Each time you bounce, you are trying to get your hands lower and lower. Although this form can help highly trained athletes who train themselves on a daily basis for a sport that has quick, herky-jerky movements, I am personally not a big fan of this method of stretching. Ballistic movements force the muscle further than it wants to go, which initiates the stretch reflex and can raise the chance of injury to muscles, tendons, and joints. I strongly urge those with bad backs and previous injuries (as well as the weekend warrior) not to use this method.

Dynamic Stretching: Most commonly used by athletes, this method of stretching involves active movements that are typically sport-specific. Mostly done with the arms and legs, and sometimes rotational stretches, dynamic stretching utilizes movements to further warm up and stretch the body's connective tissue. When done correctly, this method can be beneficial to anybody who chooses to use it. A great example would be a martial artist performing a controlled straight leg front kick to increase flexibility in the hamstring. Things to remember when performing a dynamic stretch are:

- Focus on your posture.
- Hold on to a fixed point if balance is an issue.
- Use controlled movements.
- Start slow and easy and then progress with more power (if needed).

Proprioceptive Neuromuscular Facilitation (PNF): Greater flexibility provides our body with better movement, can reduce aches and pains, improve posture, and enhance physical performance. But simply having flexibility without some kind of power from a stretched position will only hinder your functional strength. Functional strength is the ability of an individual to exert usable strength and withstand the physical force that is placed on the body. PNF is the most advanced style of stretching that is used to increase flexibility as well as strength in the muscle, which in turn gives us better functional strength.

The PNF method was originally designed to help individuals with rehab, but it has allowed trained professionals to assist people from all walks of life. The PNF method is my preferred way of stretching. It is considered by many to be the superior method in improving mobility as well as increasing strength in the stretched muscle. The downfall of this method is that it requires a trained professional to truly achieve optimal results.

One of the greatest benefits of PNF stretching is that the person being stretched can focus totally on relaxing his/her body while their partner is doing all the work. As the person is being stretched, they are then able to focus on proper breathing while also focusing on that one particular area being stretched. I have been using the PNF method of stretching for nearly two decades and have been amazed by the benefits. As I am working, I use three basic techniques:

- **Contract – Relax:** In this method, a trained professional will push or pull the muscle until a stretch is felt, holding it for approximately 10 seconds. The therapist will instruct the recipient to push back against the stretch. The recipient will then contract the muscle by pushing back against the stretch as the professional provides just enough force to allow the limb to return to the starting point. The recipient then relaxes, and the process is repeated 3-4 times.

- **Hold – Relax:** Very similar to the contract-relax method, this method uses a trained professional to push or pull the muscle until a stretch is felt, again holding the stretch for approximately 10 seconds. The recipient will be instructed to push back against the therapist, but with this method, the therapist holds the stretch for approximately 5 seconds, not allowing the recipient's body to return to the starting position. The recipient of the stretch is then asked to relax as the therapist continues to stretch the muscle. This is repeated 3-4 times before returning the body to the starting position.

- **Hold – Relax – Contract:** This method is a fantastic way to stretch, but, in my opinion, should only be done with highly trained individuals. Again, this method uses a professional who will push or pull the muscle until a stretch is felt. The recipient will then be asked to push/pull back against the stretch, which will be held for 5-10 seconds. Then the professional will instruct the recipient to pull back away from the stretch. The recipient contracts the opposite muscle getting stretched, pulling his/her body away from the professional's hand. At this point, the professional will gently push/pull the recipient's body and hold this final stretch for 5-10 seconds.

FOAM ROLLER

The foam roller can be used for myofascial release at least 2-3 times per week. Though it will be painful at first, the more often you use it (correctly, of course), the better it feels. Who knows, you may even decide to use it on a daily basis! As you use the foam roller, you are releasing tension in tight muscles (otherwise known as knots), loosening up the tension in the connective tissue between the muscles and your skin called fascia, and breaking up adhesions and scar tissue that has built up throughout your body. The best part of the foam roller is that you are in total control of the amount of pressure you place on your muscles.

Deciding when to use the foam roller depends on what you are trying to accomplish. Using it before your workout can help aid in reducing tension and increasing the range of motion in your muscles, which then helps to circulate oxygenated blood throughout the body. Using it afterward can help to re-circulate the blood that has pooled in your muscles during exercise. I love incorporating the foam roller into my stretching routines. The great thing about this piece of equipment is that you can use this at home or in your office. If you are feeling stiff or sore in a certain area, roll it out.

Before we get going into our exercises, there are a few points to remember when using the foam roller:

- Move slowly and deliberately, avoiding fast movements.
- Try to move in multiple directions. This may be difficult to accomplish if you are new to the roller, but keep working on it.
- Once you find tender areas in the muscle, hold that position for 15-30 seconds. Avoid spending too much time in one area.
- Try to get to the point where you are using it daily.
- Do not roll over your joints.

- Do not roll your lower back! The upper back is fine to work on because of the larger and stronger muscles that protect the spine. The lower back doesn't have this protection. Another thing to remember with the lower back is that just because you feel the pain there, that doesn't always mean that is the origin of the pain. Instead, focus on rolling out the muscles in your glutes and your hip flexors.

- Do not use it on an injured area, for it may cause further injury or inflammation. Instead, you can use it on the surrounding areas that may be tightening up because of the injury.

- Concentrate on your posture. Using the foam roller can be difficult as it requires you to get into some positions that utilize strength in your core and upper body. If it gets too difficult to hold the position, just come back to it.

- Use a mat or even a towel if you are on a hard floor.

- Concentrate on your breathing. Never hold your breath, as it just tightens your muscles.

FEET

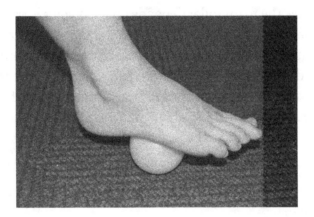

- Although this is not a foam roller, using a medium-size ball is a wonderful way to stretch and massage the muscles and tendons on the bottom of your foot. This is a great therapeutic exercise for plantar fascia and other issues causing foot pain. The use of different size balls will change the intensity of pressure on your foot. Move slowly onto the ball, making sure to not place your entire body weight on top.

CALVES

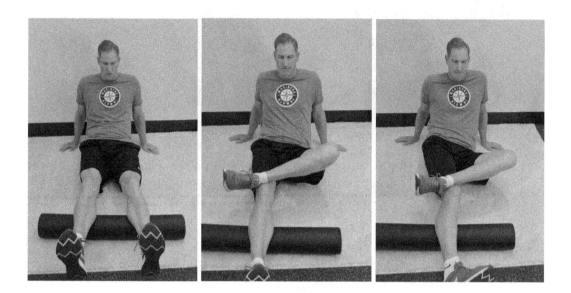

- When rolling the muscles of the calf, start in a sitting position with your hands on the ground beside you.
- Place both calves on top of the roller.
- Lift your rear off the ground and roll the length of your muscle, feeling for tenderness.
- The center picture shows an alternative way to add a little extra pressure to the muscle.
- The picture to the right shows him externally rotating his leg to roll the lateral (outside) portion of the muscle. You can do the same thing by rotating your leg medially to roll out the inside of your calf.

SHINS

- A greatly overlooked area of the body is the shins. This is a wonderful exercise for people that like to run.
- The beginner starts by simply placing their hands on the floor while placing the foam roller approximately midway up the shin.
- Roll back and forth lengthwise up the shin to find those tender areas.
- The picture on the right shows a more advanced version, which puts more pressure on the muscle.

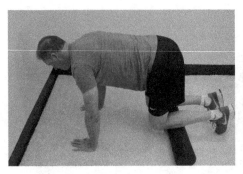 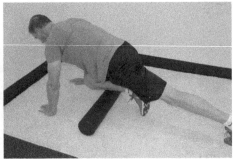

- Begin the second position by getting your hands set. Place one shin on the roller and rotate the foot so it points in and not down. Straighten out the other leg and place it behind you for stability and support.
- This position will also allow you to roll the lateral (outside) portion of the shin.

HAMSTRINGS

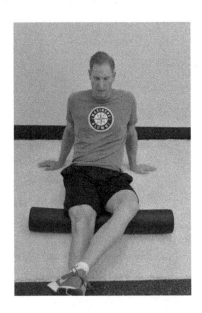

- Start by sitting on the floor with your knees slightly bent.
- Slide the foam roller underneath your legs and place it against your hamstrings (the large muscle group above the knee).
- Place your hands behind you and lift your rear off the floor.
- Slowly roll lengthwise up and down the muscle.
- Remember, when you find those tight areas, hold for 15-30 seconds.

GLUTES

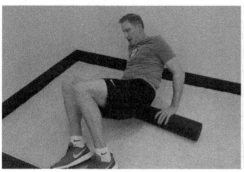 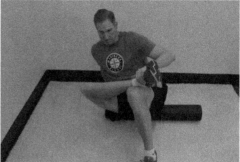

- Sit on the foam roller with your hands on the ground behind you.
- Bend both knees, keeping knees and feet together.
- Rotate your knees to the side, stabilizing yourself with the one arm that you are leaning toward. Slowly roll the muscles in your hips.
- The second picture shows the advanced version. Start by placing your right ankle on your straightened left leg, just above the knee. Ensure you are leaning on your right arm.
- Keep your ankle stabilized and bend your left knee.
- Slowly roll up and down your hip. Take note that you are now rolling a muscle that is actually getting stretched at the same time. This will be a very tender area when you first begin.

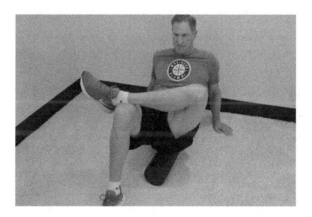

- Another great way to get into the hip is to turn the foam roller lengthwise. This will get you further into the muscles, which allow you to really work on that difficult piriformis (the piriformis is a smaller muscle in the hip that, when tight, can cause sciatic problems as well as create pain in the lower back).

- Start by sitting on the roller with both knees bent. Again, if you are rolling the left hip, lean to that side and stabilize yourself with your left arm. Roll slowly side to side.

- In the advanced version, begin by placing your left ankle on your straightened right leg, just above the knee. Ensure you are leaning on your left arm.

- Keep your ankle stabilized and bend your right knee.

- Slowly roll side to side. Again, this is working on a stretching muscle. It will be tender or even uncomfortable when you first begin.

ILIOTIBIAL BAND

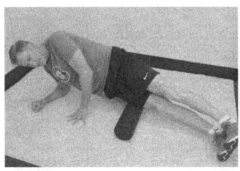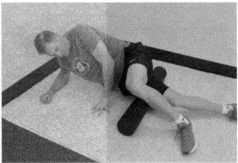

As you can guess from the name, the iliotibial band is not a muscle, but instead it is a thick band of fibrous material that we have talked about earlier called fascia. The band connects on the outside of the pelvis and runs down the outside of your leg, inserting just below your knee. Running, biking, and even weight lifting can cause tightness or inflammation of the band, sending pain down the side of your leg and into your knee.

- Start by laying the outside of your leg on the roller. In the beginning position, the leg on the roller should remain straight while the other leg is bent and the foot is resting on the ground. This position will give you more support and take some of your weight off your leg.

- In the advanced version, place your leg on top of the leg you are rolling. This will allow your own body to put more weight on the roller.

- Once you feel comfortable, slowly roll lengthwise up and down. Find those tender areas and hold for 15-30 seconds.

- Erik shows us two ways that we can place our arms. Try both positions to see what works best for you.

QUADRICEPS

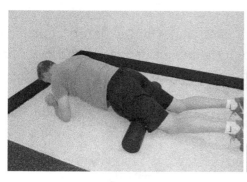 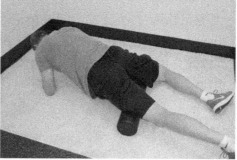

- Start off by resting on your hands and knees with the roller underneath you. Lie down with your thighs on the roller and raise your body up so you are on your elbows.
- Roll lengthwise up and down your thigh, pausing again at all those tight areas.
- The second picture shows a variation on how you can roll the different muscles in your quads. Turning your leg out will allow you to work the muscles on the inside of the thigh.

HIP FLEXORS

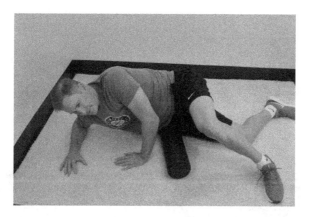

- After rolling out your quads, place the roller on the group of muscles just under your hip bone.
- If you are working on your left side, your left leg will be straight. Bend your right leg at a 90-degree angle and place your right foot on the ground. This position will give you a better base on which to move.
- While resting on your left elbow, your right hand will be on the floor, giving you more balance.

- Lean slightly to the left side and do short movements up and down your hip flexor muscles.
- This action is great for helping lower back pain. Our hip flexors attach in the front portion of our body, go through the hip and attach in the lower back. These muscles are a major cause of the inability to stand up straight after sitting for a long period of time.

ADDUCTORS

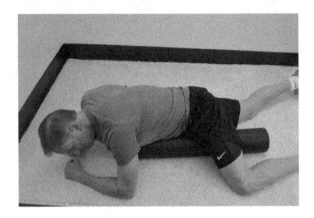

- Lie on your stomach with your elbows beneath you. Place the foam roller lengthwise to the side of you.
- Pick up your leg and place the inside of your leg on the roller.
- Slowly roll the inside of your leg lengthwise on the roller.

UPPER BACK

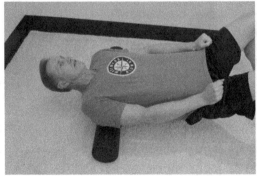 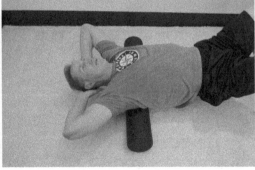

- Sit on the floor with the roller behind you and perpendicular to your body.

- Keeping your knees bent, lay back, placing the roller just above the midline.
- Raise your pelvis off the floor and slowly roll up and down your spine, ensuring that you do not take the roller lower than the rib cage.
- Relax your body and take the shape of the roller.
- The picture to the right shows a great alternative to take the pressure off your neck. This position will also allow you to round your shoulders forward.

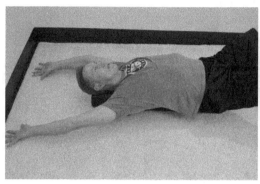 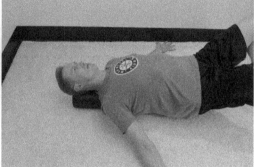

- Lie on the roller lengthwise with your head, upper back, and tailbone supported. Bend both knees and keep your feet flat on the floor for support.
- Draw your navel in and perform a pelvic tilt, laying your lower back on the roller.
- Just lying on the roller in this position with your hands on your chest may be enough.
- To add a little extra pressure to your upper back, bring your arms straight up above your head. Keep your lower back against the roller and relax.
- Now, bring your hands straight out into a T-shape position. In this position, you will feel a stretch in the upper back, chest, and the front portion of your shoulders.

LATISIMUS DORSI

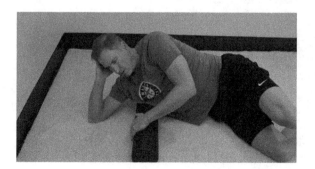

- Laying your side on the floor, place the roller underneath you just below your armpit.
- Support your head with your hand.
- Rest the leg of the side you are lying on while using your upper leg and arm to slowly move your body up and down the big muscle on the outside of your upper back.

TRICEPS

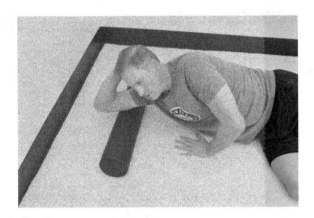

- Laying your side on the floor, place the roller underneath the back of your upper arm (triceps).
- Support your head with your hand.
- Rest the leg of the side you are lying on while using your upper leg and arm to slowly move your body up and down the length of your triceps muscle, pausing at those tender areas.

CHEST – FRONT SHOULDER

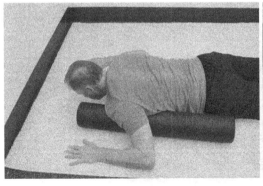 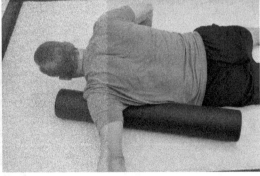

- Lying on your stomach with the roller parallel with your body, assume a modified push up position with the foam roller positioned under the armpit and shoulder.
- Slowly move outward so the roller moves in toward the chest.
- Pause when you find any tender areas.
- Men can take this through the entire area of the chest. For obvious reasons, women will have to stop short.

NECK

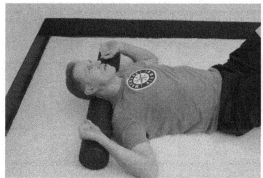 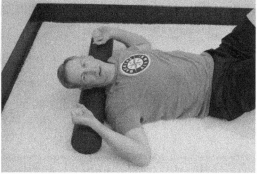

- Rolling your neck is very simple and feels great. Lying flat on your back, place the roller underneath your neck. The roller will be as close to your shoulders as possible.
- Close your eyes and just relax, taking deep breaths.
- Roll your head to the right and then to the left, pausing at any tender areas along the way.
- Place the roller on the back of your head, just above the area where your neck and head attach. You may have to play with placement to get this just right.

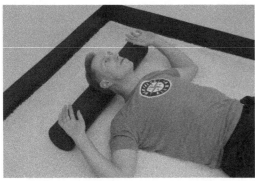 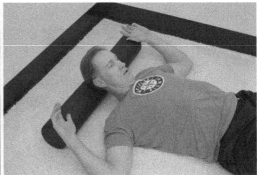

- Start by pulling the roller in toward your body with your head. Your chin should be going straight up when you do this. Hold for 3-5 seconds.

- Push the roller back out with your head. Your chin should be lowering down into your chest, stretching the back of your neck and into your upper back. Hold again and then repeat.

- As with any other stretch, some people will feel this more than others. A couple ways that you can add a little more to this stretch is by adding a pelvic tilt (rotating your hips up so your lower back is flat on the floor), or by taking your arms straight out to the side in a T-position.

SELF-EVALUATION

As great as daily stretching is, what good is it to stretch a *portion* of the body daily while neglecting other areas that may be the actual cause of your pain and discomfort? It is very important for you to understand that stretching is only as good as you make it. Whether you want to increase your flexibility for athletics or just want to loosen up rigid muscles so you don't hurt any more, you should always perform a self-evaluation. Now that we've gone over the benefits of stretching, factors affecting flexibility, and different methods of stretching, I invite you to do this self-evaluation before committing to a particular routine.

This evaluation will:

- Force you to take inventory of your own body and help to clarify any questions you may have about your own flexibility.
- Get you out of the rut of performing the same old stretches you do every day.
- Teach you what areas of the body, if tight, will create pain in other areas of the body.
- Give you a record of where you are so you can reevaluate your progress.

Before I work on anybody, I ask the following series of questions to help me determine what the individual is dealing with. On the following page, place a checkmark next to any of the following items that apply to you. By identifying these areas, you will gain an understanding not only about areas of the body that you should work on, but also areas to stay away from as well (such as areas where you have an injury to the bone or joint, pulled or torn muscle, torn ligament or tendon, and herniated or bulging discs).

MUSCULOSKELETAL: (CHECK ALL THAT APPLY)

_____ Arthritis

_____ Lower back pain

_____ Upper back pain

_____ Hip pain

_____ Injury to bone or joint

_____ Pulled or torn muscle

_____ Torn ligament or tendon

_____ Artificial joint

_____ Sciatic nerve pain

_____ Painful or swollen joints

_____ Shoulder, elbow, or wrist problems

_____ Herniated or bulging discs

On the following pages, I provide you a photo with the instructions on how to perform each stretch within the self-evaluation. I ask you to perform each stretch and circle your score below before starting any stretching routine. Doing this will allow you to understand what areas of your body move better than others and what areas need more attention. After you have your scores, work a little more diligently on those areas that are closer to number 1. With 1 meaning very little movement and 10 being great, how would you rate your range of motion in the following areas? Use the stretches that follow to help you gauge your flexibility.

• Calf	1	2	3	4	5	6	7	8	9	10
• Lower Hamstring	1	2	3	4	5	6	7	8	9	10
• Upper Hamstring	1	2	3	4	5	6	7	8	9	10
• Hips	1	2	3	4	5	6	7	8	9	10
• Inner Thigh	1	2	3	4	5	6	7	8	9	10
• Quadriceps	1	2	3	4	5	6	7	8	9	10
• Hip Flexors	1	2	3	4	5	6	7	8	9	10
• Spinal Rotation	1	2	3	4	5	6	7	8	9	10
• Shoulders	1	2	3	4	5	6	7	8	9	10
• Rotator Cuff	1	2	3	4	5	6	7	8	9	10
• Triceps	1	2	3	4	5	6	7	8	9	10
• Chest	1	2	3	4	5	6	7	8	9	10

CALF

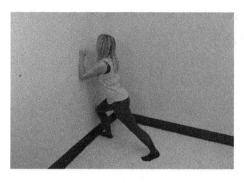

- Begin this stretch by placing the toes of one of your feet at the base of the wall.
- Placing both elbows on the wall, place your other foot a couple of feet behind you with toes pointed forward.
- Slowly lean a bit forward and down, taking your front knee and moving it toward the wall.
- Keep the heel of your back foot on the ground.
- If you can take your front knee to the wall without feeling a stretch, move your back foot back.

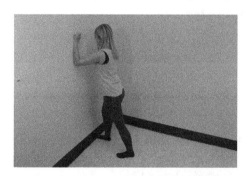

Rating of (1) Your front knee doesn't touch the wall and you are very limited on how far your back leg extends.

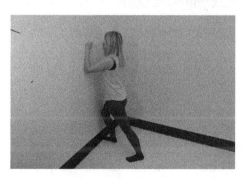

Rating of (5) Your front knee touches the wall, but you are limited on how far your back leg extends.

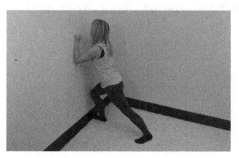

Rating of (10) Your front knee touches the wall and your leg is extended fully back, keeping your heel to the floor.

LOWER HAMSTRING

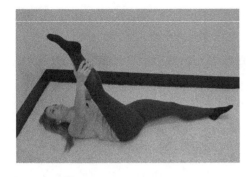

- Lie on your back, bend one knee so the bottom of your foot rests flat on the floor.
- Raise the other leg off the floor and grasp the lower portion of your calf.
- Keep your leg straight while pulling it toward you.
- Relax and hold the stretch, ensuring proper breathing.

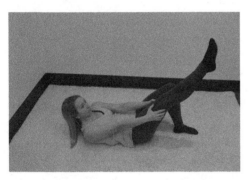

Rating of (1) You are unable to relax your head as you struggle to raise and hold your leg off the floor. You are also unable to extend your opposite leg.

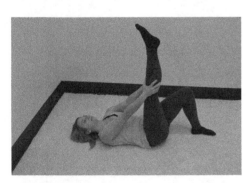

Rating of (5) Your opposite leg stays bent, but you are able to grab and pull back on your leg and relax your head back.

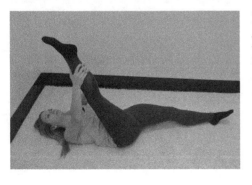

Rating of (10) You are able to fully extend your opposite leg while comfortably pulling your leg all the way back. Your head is relaxed.

UPPER HAMSTRING

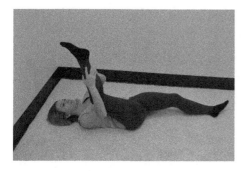

- Lie on your back with the bottom of one foot flat on the floor or bed.
- Raise your other leg off the floor and grasp the lower portion of your calf.
- With your knee bent, pull your leg down and toward your head.
- Relax and hold the stretch, ensuring proper breathing.

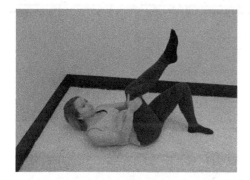

Rating of (1) You are unable to relax your head as you must grab the back of your leg to pull back. Your opposite leg remains bent.

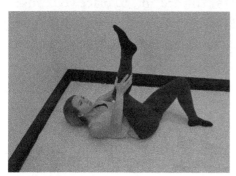

Rating of (5) You are able to pull back while grabbing your calf, but have a difficult time relaxing your head as your opposite leg is bent.

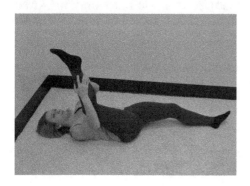

Rating of (10) You are able to fully extend your opposite leg while comfortably pulling your leg all the way back. Your head is also able to rest on the floor.

HIPS

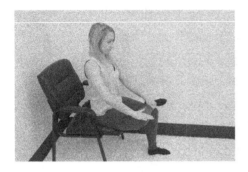

- In a seated position, place your right ankle on your left knee.
- Keeping your posture nice and tall, slowly lean forward at the hips.
- Relax and hold the stretch, ensuring proper breathing.

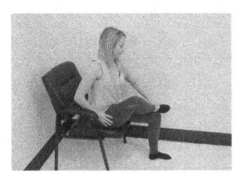

Rating of (1) You struggle to even get your ankle up on your knee. It is also very difficult to relax in this position.

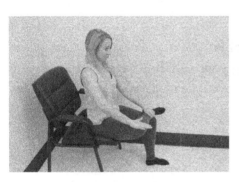

Rating of (5) You are able to place your ankle on your knee, but you feel a stretch in your hip while pushing down your knee without leaning forward.

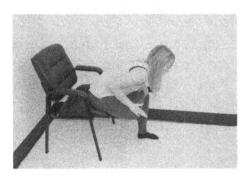

Rating of (10) Your ankle rests on your knee and you are able to lean forward, nearly touching your chest to your leg that is parallel to the floor.

INNER THIGHS

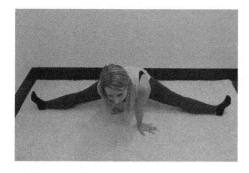

- In a standing position, slowly spread your feet apart.
- Ensuring your toes are pointed up, lower your body as far as you can (into a full split if you are able). Balance yourself by placing your hands on the floor or on another stable object.
- Relax and hold the stretch, ensuring proper breathing.

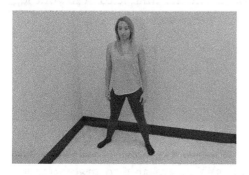

Rating of (1) You begin to feel a stretch when your feet are a little wider than shoulder width.

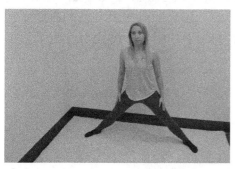

Rating of (5) You are able to get yourself halfway down to the ground as you comfortably feel the stretch.

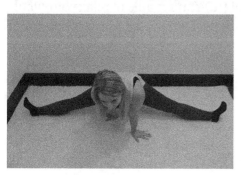

Rating of (10) You are envied by many as you comfortably go all the way down into the splits position.

QUADRICEPS

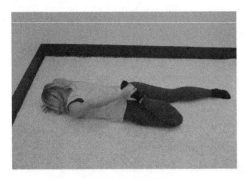

- Lie flat on your stomach.
- Pull your leg up toward your rear end and grab your ankle.
- Pull your foot in toward your rear end.
- Relax and hold the stretch, ensuring proper breathing.

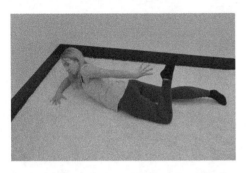

Rating of (1) You are unable to grab your leg to pull it back into your glutes.

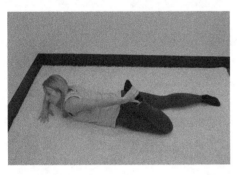

Rating of (5) You are able to grab your leg and slightly pull it down. You are unable to rest your head fully down to the ground.

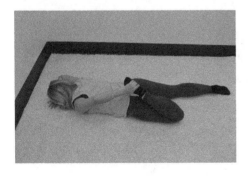

Rating of (10) You are able to relax your whole body as you pull your heel into your glutes.

HIP FLEXORS

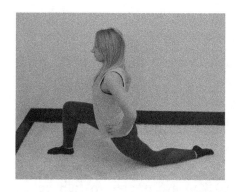

- Get down on both knees and place one foot forward in a lunge position.
- Take your weight down and forward, keeping your posture nice and tall.
- Relax and hold the stretch, ensuring proper breathing.

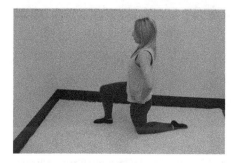

Rating of (1) You are able to get down to a knee, but you are unable to move your body down and forward toward the ground.

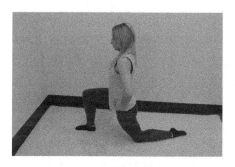

Rating of (5) You keep your forward leg in approximately a 90-degree angle as you are able to press your hip flexor down toward the ground.

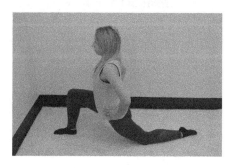

Rating of (10) Your front leg may even be at an 80- or 70- degree angle while you can nearly touch your hip flexor to the floor.

SPINAL ROTATION

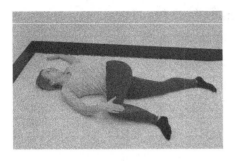

- Lie on your side, bend your top leg and place it at a 90-degree angle.
- Slowly push your top shoulder back to the ground, holding your upper knee down to the floor.
- Relax and hold the stretch, ensuring proper breathing.

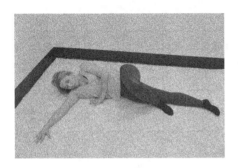

Rating of (1) You are unable to fully relax. Your head doesn't rest on the floor, your bent knee doesn't touch the floor and you are unable to lower your top shoulder down toward the floor.

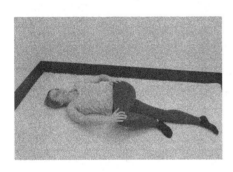

Rating of (5) You are able to relax your head to the floor. You are also able to lower your upper shoulder halfway down to the floor while slightly pulling your bent knee down toward the floor.

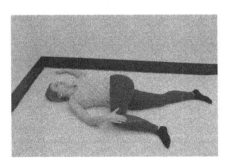

Rating of (10) You are able to fully relax your head, shoulders, and bent knee all the way down to the floor.

SHOULDERS

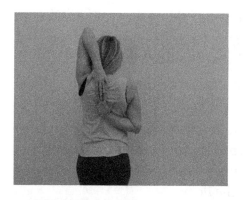

- Place one arm behind your back, and one arm bent over your head.
- Interlock your fingers and slowly pull your hands together.
- Relax and hold the stretch, ensuring proper breathing.

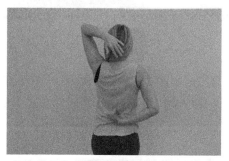

Rating of (1) You have a difficult time even getting your hands behind your back.

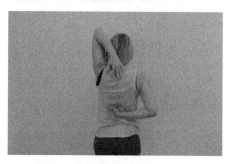

Rating of (5) Your hands are about six inches from touching.

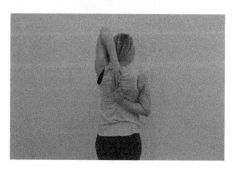

Rating of (10) You are able to lock your hands together.

ROTATOR CUFF

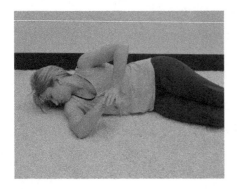

- Lying on your side, bring your arm out to a 90-degree angle. Bend your elbow and wrist also to a 90-degree angle.
- Looking straight down, place your chin on your shoulder.
- Using your other hand, grab your wrist and gently push your elbow down into the ground. Slowly push your hand down toward the floor.
- Relax and hold the stretch, ensuring proper breathing.

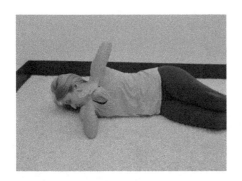

Rating of (1) You are able to get your arm and hand into a 90-degree angle, but unable to take your hand toward the ground.

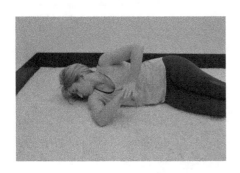

Rating of (5) With your arm and hand in a 90-degree angle, you are able to get your hand halfway down to the ground.

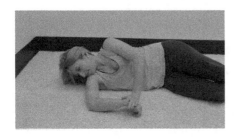

Rating of (10) After achieving the 90-degree angles, you are able to touch your fingers to the floor.

TRICEPS

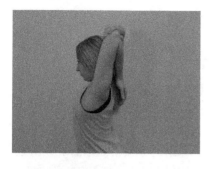

- In a standing or seated position, raise your arm over your head, bending at your elbow.
- Take your other hand and grab your elbow.
- Slowly pull your elbow back behind your head.
- Relax and hold the stretch, ensuring proper breathing.

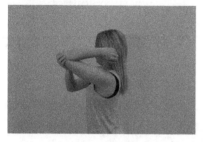

Rating of (1) You are unable to get your elbow up much higher than your shoulder.

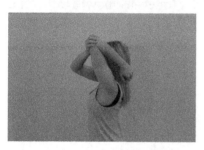

Rating of (5) You are able to get your elbow up to your head, but your arm is pointed forward.

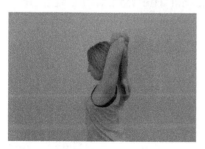

Rating of (10) You are able to get your elbow all the way up and back behind your head. Your arm is slightly pointed straight up or even slightly back.

CHEST

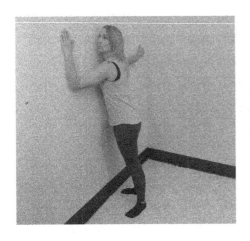

- Face a wall in a standing position.
- Place your hand, elbow, and shoulder against the wall.
- Move the opposite foot slightly away from the wall, and place your opposite palm on the wall.
- Keeping your hand, elbow, and shoulder against the wall, slowly turn your opposite shoulder away from the wall.
- Relax and hold the stretch, ensuring proper breathing.

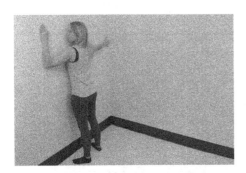

Rating of (1) You place your palm against the wall, but you are unable to rotate while keeping your shoulder (or even elbow) against the wall.

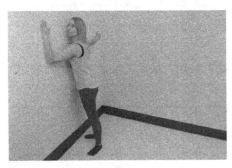

Rating of (5) You are able to keep your palm and elbow against the wall while rotating, but your shoulder begins to come away from the wall as your opposite foot steps further from the wall.

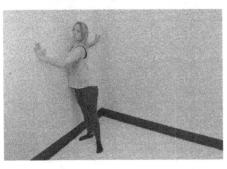

Rating of (10) You are able to stand with your side to the wall and your hand, elbow, and shoulder pressed against the wall (notice foot positions).

STATIC, PASSIVE, AND PNF STRETCHES

Whether you are a 15-year-old wannabe athlete, a 25-year-old professional athlete, a 40-year-old wondering why you are sore all the time, or an 80-year-old who has some sort of adverse physical condition, there is one thing we all want to improve: our *functional strength.*

Functional strength is the ability of an individual to exert usable strength and withstand the physical force that is placed on the body. After years of working with people from all walks of life, I understand that our main objective is to live a productive and pain-free physical lifestyle.

Whether you know it or not, functional strength either helps or prevents you from achieving your daily physical goals. It can be something that many of us take for granted, like climbing out of a chair, getting up off the ground, or even just standing upright. It can also be something that a lot of us wish we could do, like hitting the golf ball 300 yards, throwing a 95 mile-an-hour fastball, or jumping 3 feet off the ground to make a spectacular interception in the end zone. The question is, do we have the motivation and the attitude to make our functional strength grow in order to sustain it?

Lou Holtz once said that "Ability is what you're capable of doing. Motivation determines what you do. Attitude determines how well you do it."

Functional strength doesn't just come from lifting weights in a gym. It is attained through a comprehensive physical fitness program that works on *all* aspects of physical movement. Weight training plays a key role, but if you aren't working on your flexibility as well, you are missing a key component in your overall well-being. The stretches within this book were compiled to give you multiple options so that you can choose those that best fit your personal needs. They have been grouped together by difficulty and muscle group, but understand that many of the stretches can (and will) be felt in other areas of the body as well.

I have also separated the stretches into two different sections, with the first being static and passive stretches. As you go through this section, remember that passive stretching utilizes an outside force such as a partner, straps, a towel, or a machine like a cable crossover, whereas static stretches are different poses and positions you get your body into to feel a stretch. I would prefer you do these stretches after your workout, not before, or even on days off after your warm-up.

The second section is dynamic stretches. I mentioned earlier in the book that dynamic stretches are typically done by athletes, which is true, but I am really making a push for my clients to add it to their daily exercise and stretching routine, and I urge you to do the same. Dynamic stretches involve active movements to stretch the muscle. They may be more of a workout than a nice relaxing stretch for some of you, but this is also why I want you to do them. Add these in after your warm-up and before your workout to get the most out of your muscles. You can also do these on a daily basis, even if you are not planning to work out.

As you go through the stretches that follow, take note that I have separated the stretches into three different categories: **Anyone**, **Intermediate**, and **Advanced**. When deciding on what stretches you should incorporate, I strongly suggest that you utilize your self-evaluation. If your score falls between 1-4, I suggest using the stretches that **Anyone** can do. Scores between 5-7 should focus on the **Intermediate** and also the stretches that **Anyone** can do. For those of you with a score of 8-10, you can also add in the **Advanced** stretches.

Please note that many stretches are advanced and can be dangerous for some people to try. Some stretches also utilize equipment, such as a T-Stretch strap, a ball, or even weights. My desire to write this book was to give everybody a wide variety of stretches to incorporate into their daily lives. Before you start your program, there are a few things you want to do:

- Consult a physician before beginning.
- Warm up for at least 5-10 minutes.
- Take stretching seriously! Focus on what you are trying to accomplish.
- Focus on posture. You should sit or stand nice and tall, no slouching.

- Move slowly in and out of each stretch.
- Focus on proper breathing. As you breathe in, focus on that oxygen going to the muscle you are stretching.
- Be comfortable when stretching. Wear loose-fitting or stretchy clothes.
- Consciously focus on the muscle being stretched.
- If you are performing a static or passive stretch, hold the stretch for at least 20-30 seconds.
- Get rid of all distractions. Find a quiet place to stretch.

STATIC AND PASSIVE STRETCHES

Static and passive are the two most widely used forms of stretching that people use today. Both methods are easy to perform and are typically a little more relaxing. I encourage you to take advantage of these two methods *after* your workout. Always remember that a warm muscle is easier and safer to stretch than a cold one. If you decide that you would like to stretch and you haven't worked out, I would still encourage you to perform a 5- to 10-minute warm-up. A few key points to remember are:

- Focus on your breathing.
- Use a foam roller to help release adhesions in the muscles.
- Ensure proper posture
- Find a relaxing area to stretch.
- Concentrate on fully relaxing your body.
- Hold each stretch for at least 20-30 seconds, but don't be afraid to hold it for several minutes as long as you feel comfortable.

ANKLES, FEET, AND SHINS

When you make your decision to stretch, how many of your stretches are focused on your ankles, feet, or shins? Most people don't even think about stretching these areas unless they have some sort of problem, and trust me—you don't want to have those problems! Some common issues that can arise are:

- Arthritis
- Shin splints
- Plantar Fasciitis

- Tight Achilles tendon
- Ankle sprains
- Dropped arches (which can cause your foot to roll in)

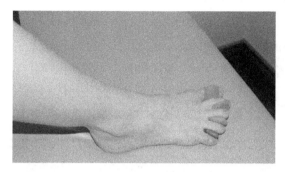

- Place smooth rocks or spacers in between your toes.
- I particularly like doing this with the rocks warmed. You can accomplish this by placing the rocks in hot water. Just ensure that the rocks are not too hot.

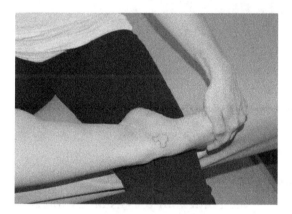

- Sitting in an upright position, place your ankle on your knee.
- Grasp your toes at the top of the foot and slowly pull your toes down.
- Hold the stretch, relax, and ensure proper breathing.

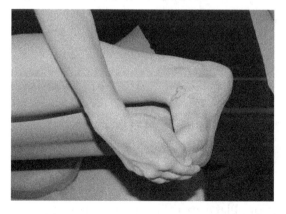

- Sitting in an upright position, place your ankle on your knee.
- Grasp underneath your toes and slowly pull your toes up.
- Hold the stretch, relax, and ensure proper breathing.

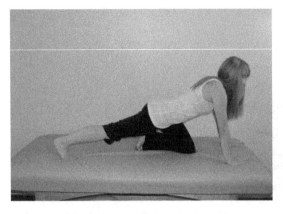

- Start this stretch from your hands and knees.
- Take one leg straight back and place toes on the floor.
- Slowly lean back into your back foot.
- Though you may feel this in your calf as well, ensure that you are focusing on stretching the bottom of the foot.
- Hold the stretch, relax, and ensure proper breathing.

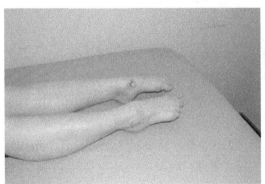 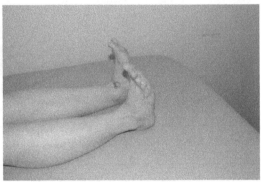

- You can perform this simple dynamic stretch sitting on the floor or in a chair.
- With your legs straight out in front of you, point your toes as far as you can, hold for a second or two, and then pull your toes toward you as far as you can.
- Relax and repeat this 10-15 times, ensuring proper breathing.

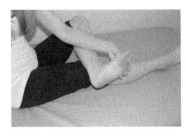 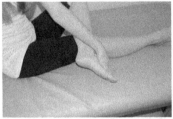 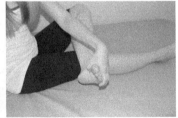

- Start off this stretch in a sitting position. Place an ankle on top of the opposite knee.
- Take hold of your foot and rotate your foot in a large circle.

- This stretch will take some time to learn how to do it properly. Many people want to help rotate the foot with the muscles that are supposed to be relaxed.
- Work on relaxing those muscles around your ankle while you manually rotate your foot.
- Relax and repeat this 10-15 times, ensuring proper breathing.

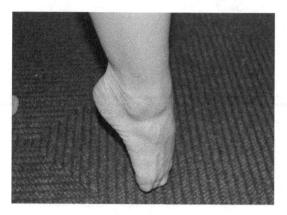

- Standing up with one leg slightly in front of the other, curl your toes under your foot.
- Very gently lean forward and push down and into your foot.
- Hold the stretch, relax, and ensure proper breathing.
- Do not do this stretch if you have balance issues. **(Intermediate)**

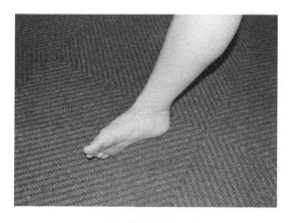

- Standing up with one leg slightly in front of the other, rotate on the outside of your foot.
- Slowly push down and feel the stretch on the outside of the foot and ankle.
- Hold the stretch, relax and ensure proper breathing.
- Do not do if you have balance issues. **(Intermediate)**

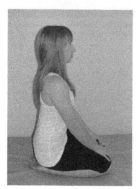

- Start this position on your knees with your toes pointed backward.
- Slowly sit down on your heels.
- Relax and hold this position, ensuring proper breathing.

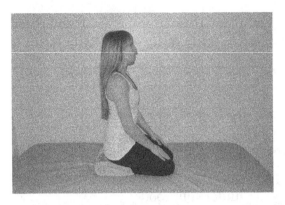

- The second picture shows an even more advanced version of this stretch with a towel placed under her feet. **(Intermediate)**

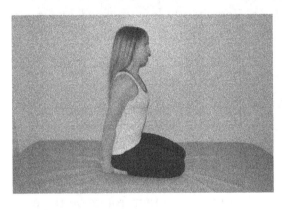

- A third and even more advanced version of this stretch has her sitting on her feet.
- She then reaches back to pull her toes up.
- Relax and hold the position. **(Advanced)**

CALVES

Do you remember that children's song about how your thigh bone is connected to your hip bone? I actually use this song when I talk to people about the human body because it works that way with our muscles as well. Just because you feel pain in one area doesn't necessarily mean that is where the problem is. The calf is a great example of how tightness in one area may affect other areas of the body as well. Some common problems with tight calves are:

- Calf pain
- Foot and heel pain
- Plantar fasciitis
- Problems with the Achilles tendon
- Knee pain
- Shin splints
- Pain up into the hamstrings, glutes (hip), and even lower back

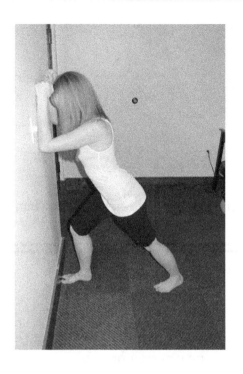

- Begin this stretch by placing the toes of one of your feet at the base of the wall.
- Placing both elbows on the wall, place your other foot a couple of feet behind you with toes pointed forward.
- Slowly lean a bit forward and down, taking your front knee and moving it toward the wall.
- Keep the heel of your back foot on the ground.
- If you can take your front knee to the wall without feeling a stretch, move your back foot back.
- Relax and hold the stretch, ensuring proper breathing.

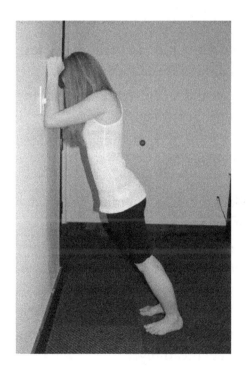

- Standing approximately an arm's length away from the wall, stand with your feet about six inches apart with toes pointed forward.
- Lean on the wall with both elbows. Ensure that you keep a straight line with your knees, hips, back, and neck. Do not let your hips sink in toward the wall.
- Stand with both heels on the ground.
- If your heels are on the ground and you do not feel a stretch, move back.
- Relax and hold the stretch, ensuring proper breathing.

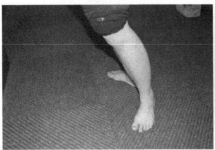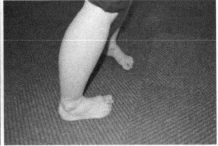

- These two pictures show a couple of different ways to position your feet when doing the previous stretch.
- Turn feet out or in before leaning into the wall to stretch a totally different area in the calf.
- Relax and hold the stretch, ensuring proper breathing.

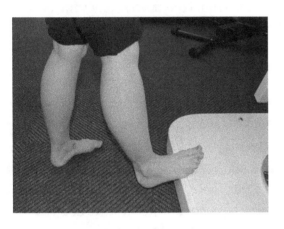

- Place the ball of your foot on the edge of any type of riser or step.
- Keeping your leg straight, slowly push the heel of your foot down. Keeping your body nice and tall, slowly lean forward to enhance the stretch.
- Relax and hold the stretch, ensuring proper breathing.
- Hold on to something for added balance.

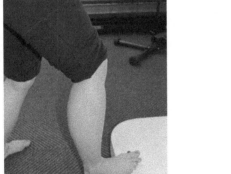

- Place the ball of your foot on the edge of any riser or step.
- Bend your knee slightly and slowly push the heel of your foot down. Keeping your body nice and tall, slowly lean forward to enhance the stretch.
- Relax and hold the stretch, ensuring proper breathing.
- Hold on to something for added balance.

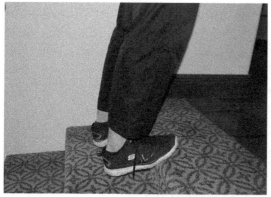

- Standing with your body nice and tall, place the balls of your feet on the edge of any riser or step.
- Keeping both legs straight, slowly lower both heels toward the ground.
- Relax and hold the stretch, ensuring proper breathing.
- Hold on to something for added balance.

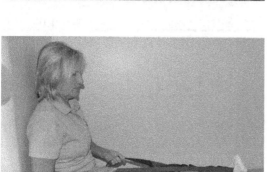

- Sit with both legs straight in front of you.
- Place a strap or towel around the ball of your foot (just below your toes).
- Relax your foot and pull the strap back.
- Relax and hold the stretch, ensuring proper breathing.
- You may also want to sit against the wall for added support.

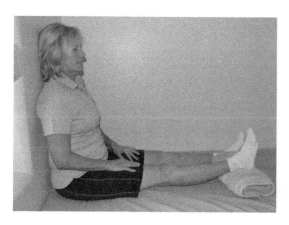

- Sit with both legs straight in front of you.
- Place a rolled-up towel under your heel.
- Relax your leg so that the back of your knee lowers toward the floor.
- Relax and hold the stretch, ensuring proper breathing.
- You may also want to sit against the wall for added support.

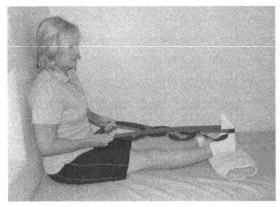

- Sitting with both legs straight in front of you, place a rolled-up towel under your heel.
- Place a strap or towel around the ball of your foot (just below your toes).
- Relax your foot and pull the strap back.
- Relax and hold the stretch, ensuring proper breathing.
- Sitting against the wall will give you some added support.

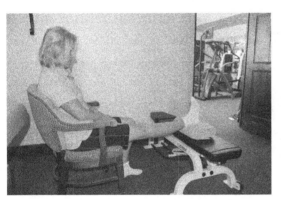

- Sit in a chair with another chair or stationary object in front of you. Place a rolled-up towel on the chair in front of you.
- Put your foot on top of the towel and relax your knee down toward the ground.
- Relax and hold the stretch, ensuring proper breathing.

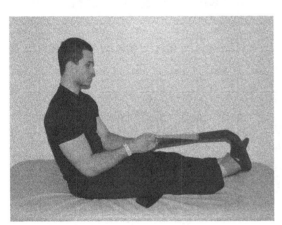

- In a seated position, place the T-Stretch strap around your ankle and up the bottom of your foot.
- Keeping your posture nice and tall, relax your foot and pull the strap toward you.
- Relax and hold the stretch, ensuring proper breathing.

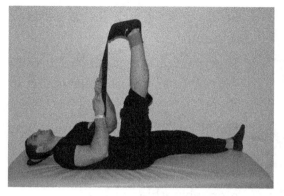

- Lying flat on your back, place the T-Stretch strap around your ankle and up the bottom of your foot.
- Bring your leg straight up and pull back and down on the strap.
- Relax and hold the stretch, ensuring proper breathing.

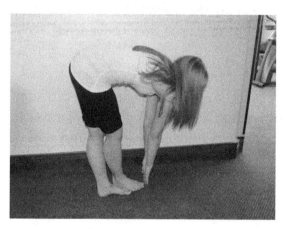

- In a standing position, cross one leg in front of the other.
- Keeping your posture nice and tall (try not to arch the back), bend forward at the hips. This move will give you an intense stretch behind the knee.
- Relax and hold the stretch, ensuring proper breathing. Slowly rise up when you are done. **(Intermediate)**

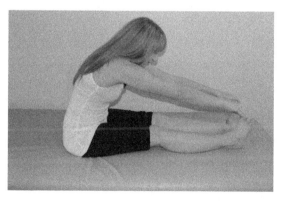

- Sit with both legs straight in front of you.
- Keeping your posture nice and tall, bend forward at the hips and grab your toes.
- Pull toes back.
- Relax and hold the stretch, ensuring proper breathing. **(Advanced)**

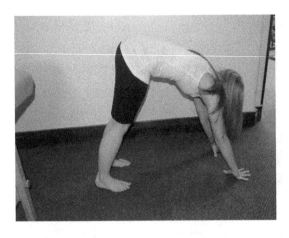

- Begin this stretch in a push-up position.
- Slowly move your hands back toward your feet and lift your hips higher in the air.
- Slowly push your heels back into the ground.
- Relax and hold the stretch, ensuring proper breathing.
- End the stretch by returning to a push-up position. **(Advanced)**

HAMSTRINGS

The hamstrings consist of three muscles that, when tight, can be the cause of a number of problems. Whether you realize it or not, our hamstrings play a major role in how we move daily. Whether you are a martial arts student trying to improve your front kicks, or if you are someone just trying to improve the length of your stride when you walk, you want to focus on stretching these three muscles. Common problems associated with tight hamstrings are:

- Arthritic pain
- Knee pain
- Hip pain
- Back pain
- Sacroiliac joint pain (located at the bottom of the spine)
- Poor posture

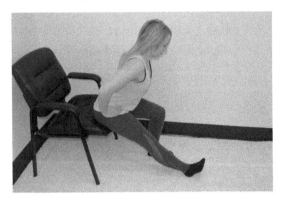

- Sit toward the end of a chair with one leg bent and the other leg straight out with the heel on the floor.
- Keeping your posture nice and tall, bend forward at the hips until you reach a stretched position. Do not hunch your back.
- Relax and hold the stretch, ensuring proper breathing.

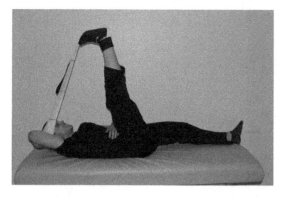

- Lying on your back, place the T-Stretch strap around your ankle and up the bottom of your foot.
- Keeping your leg straight, pull your leg toward you.
- Relax and hold the stretch, ensuring proper breathing.

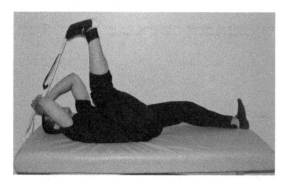

- Lying on your back, place the T-Stretch strap around your ankle and under the bottom of your foot.
- With your knee bent, pull leg down and toward your head.
- Relax and hold the stretch, ensuring proper breathing.

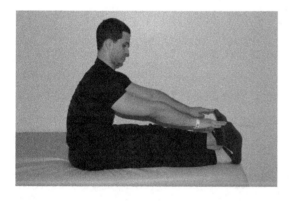

- Sit with your legs straight out in front of you.
- Keeping your posture nice and tall, bend forward at the hips until you reach a stretched position. Do not hunch your back.
- Relax and hold the stretch, ensuring proper breathing.

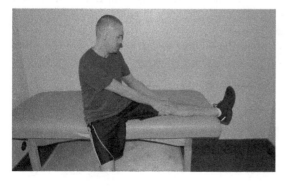

- Sit on the edge of your bed or table.
- Place one leg straight out on the table and the other leg on the floor for balance.
- Keeping your posture nice and tall, bend forward at the hips until you reach a stretched position. Do not hunch your back.
- Relax and hold the stretch, ensuring proper breathing.

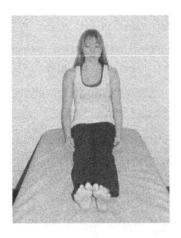

- Sit with your back flat against the wall.
- Place your legs together, straight out in front of you.
- Keeping your posture nice and tall, move your rear end toward the wall.
- Relax and hold the stretch, ensuring proper breathing.

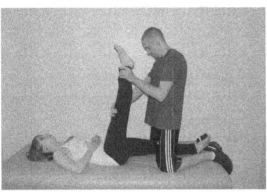

- While lying on your back, have your partner pick one leg up, placing one hand just above the knee on your thigh and the other hand just above your heel.
- Keeping your leg straight, have your partner slowly push your leg back until the stretch is felt.
- Relax and hold the stretch, ensuring proper breathing.

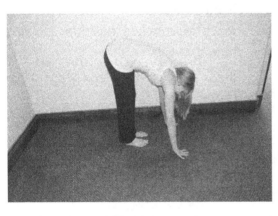

- Stand with both feet together.
- Keeping your posture nice and tall, bend forward at the hips. Do not hunch your back.
- With this stretch, you can let your arms hang, place them on the back of your head, or grab your calves.
- Relax and hold the stretch, ensuring proper breathing.

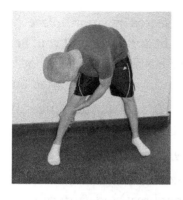

- Stand with your legs straight and a little wider than shoulder-width apart.
- Keeping your posture nice and tall, bend forward at the hips toward the right side.
- Grasp behind the leg and pull down slightly.
- Relax and hold the stretch, ensuring proper breathing.

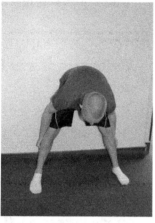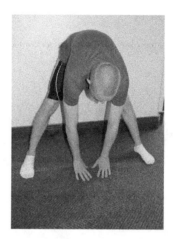

- Stand with your legs straight and feet a little wider than shoulder-width apart.
- Keeping a nice tall posture, bend forward at the hips.
- If you are unable to touch the floor, grasp behind your legs and hold.
- If you are able to touch the floor, work on placing your palms on the floor (don't force it).
- Relax and hold the stretch, ensuring proper breathing.
- Bad backs beware. **(Intermediate)**

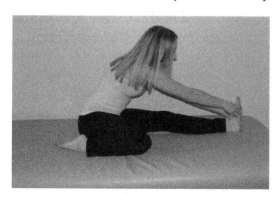

- In a seated position, place one leg straight out in front of you. Bend the other leg and place the foot behind you.
- Keeping your posture nice and tall, bend forward at the hips.
- Slowly reach for your toes.
- Relax and hold the stretch, ensuring proper breathing. **(Intermediate)**

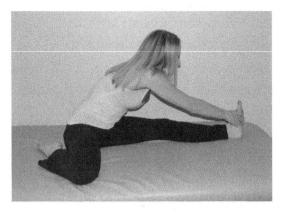

- In a seated position, place one leg straight out in front of you. Bend the other leg and place the foot behind you with your knee pointed out.
- Keeping your posture nice and tall, bend forward at the hips.
- Slowly reach for your toes.
- Relax and hold the stretch, ensuring proper breathing. **(Intermediate)**

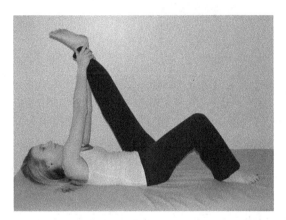

- Lie on your back, bend one knee so the bottom of your foot rests flat on the floor.
- Raise the other leg off the floor and grasp the lower portion of your calf.
- Keep your leg straight while pulling it toward you.
- Relax and hold the stretch, ensuring proper breathing. **(Intermediate)**

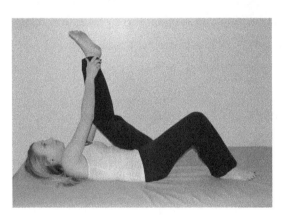

- Lie on your back with the bottom of one foot flat on the floor or bed.
- Raise your other leg off the floor and grasp the lower portion of your calf.
- With your knee bent, pull your leg down and toward your head.
- Relax and hold the stretch, ensuring proper breathing. **(Intermediate)**

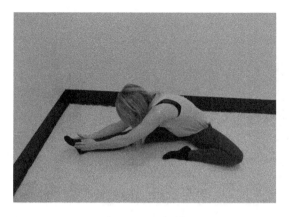

- In a seated position, straighten one leg and place it out into a splits position. Bend your other leg and bring your foot in close to your body.
- Keeping your posture nice and tall, bend toward the straightened leg.
- Relax and hold the stretch, ensuring proper breathing. **(Intermediate)**

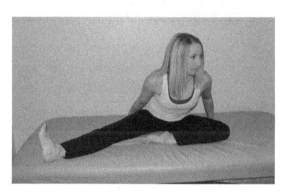

- In a seated position, straighten one leg and place it out in a splits position. Bend your other leg and bring your foot in close to your body.
- Keeping your posture nice and tall, bend forward.
- Relax and hold the stretch, ensuring proper breathing. **(Intermediate)**

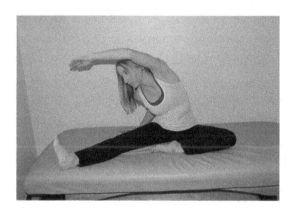

- In a seated position, straighten one leg and place it out in a splits position. Bend your other leg and bring your foot in close to your body.
- Straighten both arms above your head.
- Keeping your posture nice and tall, perform a side bend toward the straightened leg.
- Relax and hold the stretch, ensuring proper breathing. **(Intermediate)**

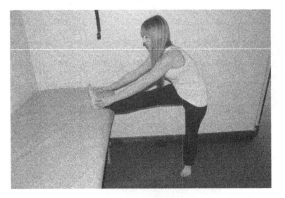

- Place your foot on a stationary object. The more flexibility you have, the higher you can place your foot.
- Keeping your back straight, lean toward your foot.
- Relax and hold the stretch, ensuring proper breathing. **(Intermediate)**

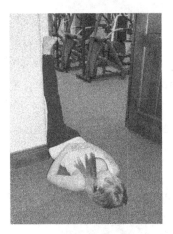

- Lying on the floor, position yourself near a doorway.
- Place the leg you would like to stretch up the edge of the wall and your other leg through the doorway.
- Move your body toward the doorway until you feel the stretch.
- Relax and hold the stretch, ensuring proper breathing. **(Advanced)**

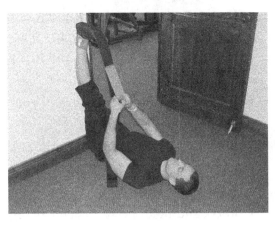

- Lying on the floor, position yourself near a doorway.
- Place the leg you would like to stretch up the edge of the wall and your other leg through the doorway. Move your body toward the wall until the stretch is felt.
- Place a T-Stretch strap over the ball of your foot and pull your toes down.
- Relax and hold the stretch, ensuring proper breathing. **(Advanced)**

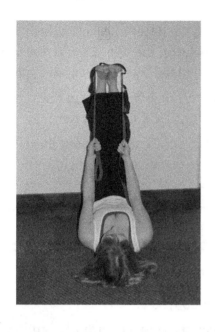

- Lying on your back, place both legs straight up on a wall.
- Move your body as close to the wall as you can. The goal is to eventually get your rear end to the wall.
- Place a strap over the balls of both feet and pull down.
- Relax and hold the stretch, ensuring proper breathing.
- Ensure that your rear end and lower back do not come off the floor. Move away from the wall until you are flat on the ground. **(Advanced)**

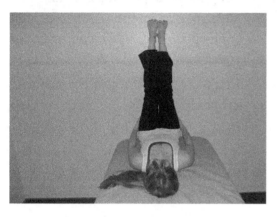

- Lying on your back, place both legs straight up the wall.
- Slowly move your body in toward the wall until the stretch is felt.
- Relax and hold the stretch, ensuring proper breathing.
- Ensure that your rear end and lower back do not rise off the floor. Move back in order to lie flat on the floor. **(Advanced)**

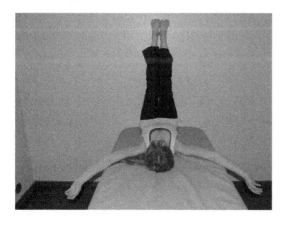

- Lying on your back, place both legs straight up the wall, ensure that your rear end and lower back stay on the floor.
- Slowly move your body in toward the wall until the stretch is felt. You will feel this in your hamstrings and possibly even your mid back.
- Place both arms straight out on the floor.
- Relax and hold the stretch, ensuring proper breathing. **(Advanced)**

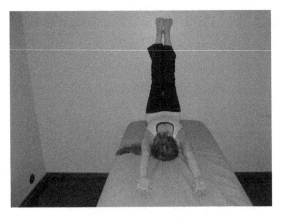

- Lying on your back, place both legs straight up the wall. Ensure that your rear end and lower back stay on the floor.
- Slowly move your body in toward the wall until the stretch is felt.
- Reach both arms over your head. You may feel this stretch in your mid- to upper back as well.
- Relax and hold the stretch, ensuring proper breathing. **(Advanced)**

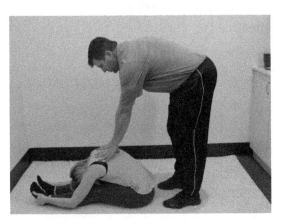

- Sit with your legs straight out in front of you.
- Keeping your posture nice and tall, have your partner GENTLY push on your upper back while you reach for your toes.
- Relax and hold the stretch, ensuring proper breathing.
- Communicate with your partner, letting him/her know when you feel the stretch. **(Advanced)**

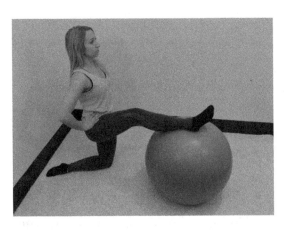

- Place your heel on the center of the ball and lower yourself so your other knee is on the ground (use a wall or other stationary object for support if necessary).
- Keep your leg slightly bent and your posture nice and tall. Slowly move the ball toward you.
- Relax and hold the stretch, ensuring proper breathing. **(Advanced)**

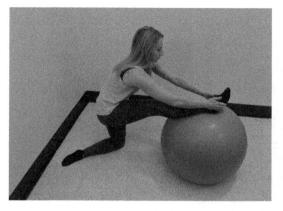

- Place your heel on the center of the ball and lower yourself so your other knee is on the ground (use a wall or other stationary object for support if necessary).
- Keeping your leg slightly bent and your posture nice and tall, slowly bend down to grab your foot.
- Relax and hold the stretch, ensuring proper breathing. **(Advanced)**

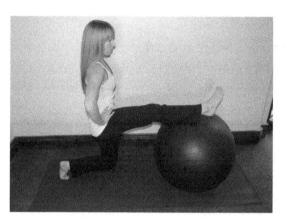

- Place your heel on the center of the ball and lower yourself so your other knee is on the ground (use a wall or other stationary object for support if necessary).
- Focus on keeping your leg straight while keeping your posture nice and tall.
- Relax and hold the stretch, ensuring proper breathing. **(Advanced)**

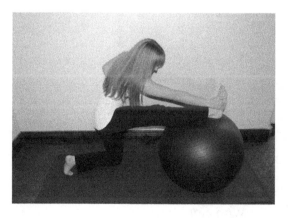

- Place your heel on the center of the ball and lower yourself so your other knee is on the ground (use a wall or other stationary object for support if necessary).
- Focusing on keeping your leg straight and your posture nice and tall, slowly lean forward to reach for your foot.
- Relax and hold the stretch, ensuring proper breathing. **(Advanced)**

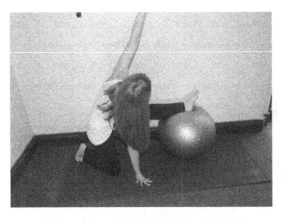

- Place your heel on the center of the ball and lower yourself so your other knee is on the ground (use a wall or other stationary object for support if necessary).
- Focus on keeping your leg straight while leaning to the other side.
- Place your opposite hand on the floor while reaching to the sky with your other arm.
- Relax and hold the stretch, ensuring proper breathing. **(Advanced)**

ADDUCTORS

There is a common misconception, primarily among men, that the hip adductors don't need work. I have heard all sorts of excuses, anything from, "I am not in karate" to, "That is only for women." I am sorry to burst your bubble, men, but this muscle group is not only important for everyday actions, such as walking, but tight or weak hip adductors can cause:

- Arthritic pain
- Knee pain
- Hip pain
- Lower back pain
- Decreased circulation down the leg

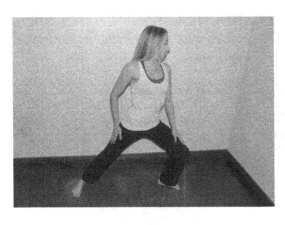

- In a standing position, spread your legs approximately three feet apart.
- Keeping your right foot pointed forward, turn your left foot out to the side.
- Keeping your posture nice and tall, lunge to the left side and push down with right hip.
- Relax and hold the position, ensuring proper breathing.

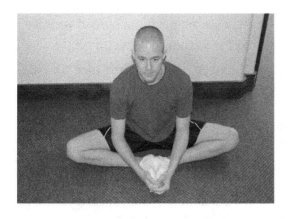

- In a seated position, bend your knees and bring the bottoms of your feet together.
- Sitting nice and tall, pull your feet in close to your body.
- Let your knees lay down to the ground.
- Relax and hold the position, ensuring proper breathing.

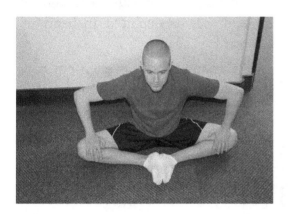

- In a seated position, bend your knees and bring the bottoms of your feet together.
- Sitting nice and tall, pull your feet in close to your body.
- Let your knees relax down to the ground and slowly push down on your knees.
- Relax and hold position, ensuring proper breathing.

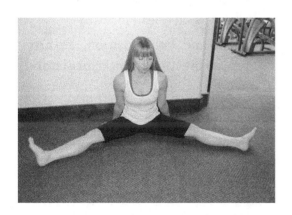

- Start in a seated position, keeping your posture nice and tall.
- Spread your legs as far as they will let you go.
- If you have a tendency to want to lean back, sit with your back against a wall to keep you from rocking back.
- Relax and hold the stretch, ensuring proper breathing.

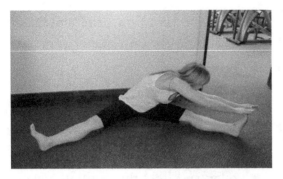

- In a seated position, spread your legs as far as they will let you go.
- Keeping your posture nice and tall and your toes pointed up, bend to one side.
- Relax and hold the stretch, ensuring proper breathing. **(Intermediate)**

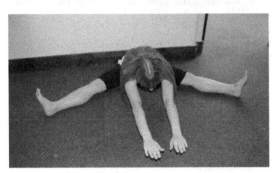

- In a seated position, spread your legs as far as they will go.
- Keeping your posture nice and tall and your toes pointed up, bend forward at the hips.
- Relax and hold the stretch, ensuring proper breathing. **(Intermediate)**

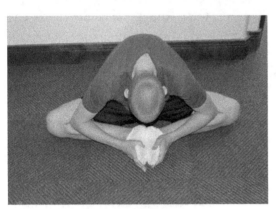

- In a seated position, bend your knees and bring the bottoms of your feet together.
- Pull your feet in close to your body.
- Let your knees lay down to the ground. Pushing your knees down with your elbows, slowly lean forward.
- Relax and hold position, ensuring proper breathing. **(Intermediate)**

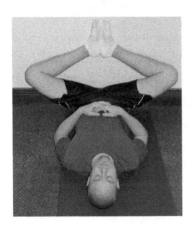

- Lie on your back on the floor, pull yourself in toward the wall. Straighten your legs up the wall.
- Bend your knees and bring the bottoms of your feet together.
- Pull your feet down the wall toward your hips.
- Relax and hold the position, ensuring proper breathing.

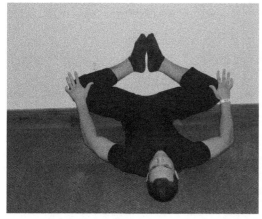

- Lie on your back on the floor and pull yourself in toward the wall. Straighten your legs up the wall.
- Bend your knees and bring the bottoms of your feet together.
- Pull your feet down the wall toward your hips and slowly push your knees in toward the wall.
- Relax and hold the position, ensuring proper breathing. **(Intermediate)**

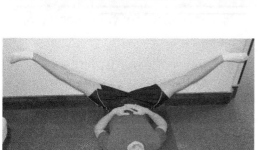

- Lie on your back on the floor, pulling yourself in toward the wall. Straighten your legs up the wall.
- Slowly lower your legs out to the side.
- Relax and hold the position, ensuring proper breathing. **(Intermediate)**

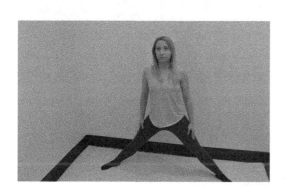

- In a standing position, slowly spread your feet apart until you feel the stretch in between your legs.
- Keep your posture nice and tall.
- Relax and hold the position, ensuring proper breathing.
- This stretch puts pressure on the inside of your knees. Do not perform this stretch if you have bad or unstable knees. **(Intermediate)**

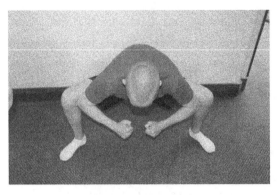

- Stand with your feet approximately three feet apart.
- Squat down, keeping your knees above your heels.
- Place your elbows on the inside of your knees and push out.
- Relax and hold the stretch, ensuring proper breathing. **(Intermediate)**

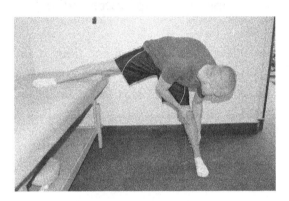

- Place the inside of your foot on top of a bed or table.
- Keeping your posture nice and tall, slowly bend down toward your foot on the ground.
- Relax and hold the stretch, ensuring proper breathing. **(Intermediate)**

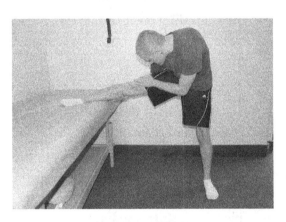

- Place the inside of your foot on top of your bed or table.
- Keeping your posture nice and tall, slowly lean into your top leg.
- Relax and hold the stretch, ensuring proper breathing. **(Intermediate)**

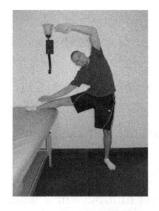

- Place the inside of your foot on top of your bed or table.
- Stretch your arms above your head and slowly perform a side bend toward your top leg.
- Relax and hold the stretch, ensuring proper breathing. **(Intermediate)**

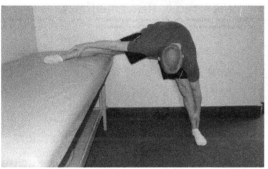

- Place the inside of your foot on top of your bed or table.
- Keeping your posture nice and tall, slowly bend down at the hips, grabbing both ankles.
- Relax and hold the stretch, ensuring proper breathing. **(Intermediate)**

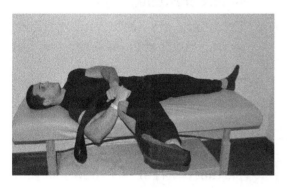

- Place a T-Stretch strap around your foot and lie flat on your back.
- Take your leg as far out to the side as you can.
- Using one arm, pull on the strap, pulling your leg out even further.
- Relax and hold the stretch, ensuring proper breathing. **(Intermediate)**

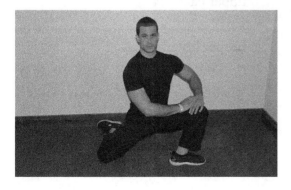

- Get down on both knees. Bend your left knee and place it out so your knee and toes are pointed to the side.
- Slowly take your weight to the left side and push your groin down toward the ground.
- Relax and hold the stretch, ensuring proper breathing. **(Intermediate)**

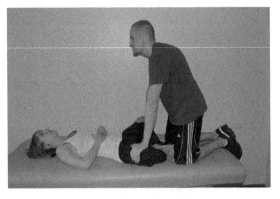

- Lying on your back, place the bottom of your feet together and relax your knees out.
- Have your partner GENTLY push your knees down toward the table.
- Relax and hold the stretch, ensuring proper breathing.
- Communicate with your partner, letting him/her know when you feel the stretch. **(Intermediate)**

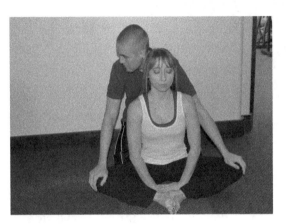

- In a seated position, place the bottom of your feet together and relax your knees out.
- Have your partner GENTLY push your knees down toward the floor.
- Relax and hold the stretch, ensuring proper breathing.
- Communicate with your partner, letting him/her know when you feel the stretch. **(Intermediate)**

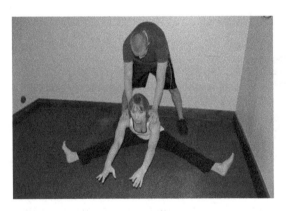

- In a seated position, spread your legs as far out as they can go.
- Keeping your posture tall, have your partner GENTLY push down on your upper back.
- Relax and hold the stretch, ensuring proper breathing.
- Communicate with your partner, letting him/her know when you feel the stretch. **(Advanced)**

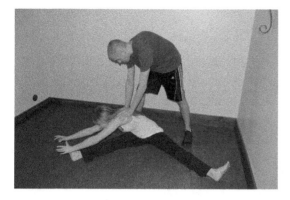

- In a seated position, spread your legs as far out as they will go.
- While trying to avoid hunching over, reach down toward your foot. Have your partner GENTLY push down on your upper back.
- Relax and hold the stretch, ensuring proper breathing.
- Communicate with your partner, letting him/her know when you feel the stretch. **(Advanced)**

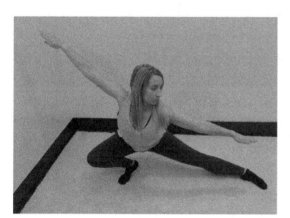

- Spread your legs approximately twice your shoulder width.
- Squat down on the right side, keeping your left leg straight.
- Keeping your arms in a straight line with your left leg, slowly push the inside of your left leg to the ground.
- Relax and hold the stretch, ensuring proper breathing. **(Advanced)**

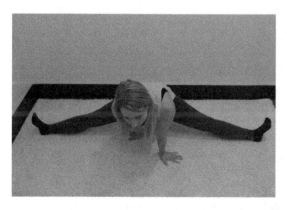

- In a standing position, slowly spread your feet apart.
- Ensuring your toes are pointed up, lower your body as far as you can (into a full split if you are able). Balance yourself by placing your hands on the floor or other stable object.
- Relax and hold the stretch, ensuring proper breathing. **(Advanced)**

THIGHS AND HIP FLEXORS

Everything we do on a daily basis can tighten our muscles, creating pain all over our bodies. Whether you are a hiker, biker, or an office worker who sits behind a desk all day, you are at risk of suffering from tight thighs and hip flexors. Some common problems that can occur are:

- Arthritic pain
- Poor posture
- Knee pain
- Hip pain
- Lower back pain

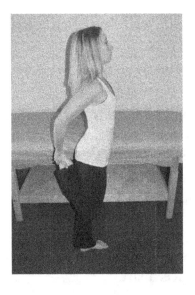

- Stand with both feet together, keeping your posture nice and tall.
- Pick one leg up behind you, reach around and grab your foot.
- Pull your knee in toward your rear end. Try not to let your knee move forward.
- Keep your posture nice and tall, not letting your shoulder slump forward.
- Relax and hold the stretch, ensuring proper breathing.
- If you have trouble keeping balanced, hold on to something sturdy.

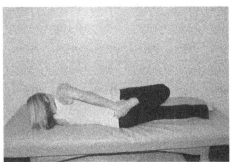

- Lie on your side.
- Bring one leg back and grab it with your hand.
- Pull your knee in toward your rear end, keeping it from moving forward.
- Keep your body from tipping forward.
- Relax and hold the stretch, ensuring proper breathing.

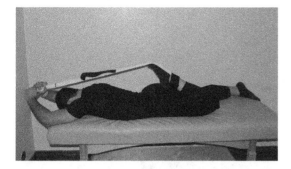

- Place a T-Stretch strap around your foot and lie flat on your stomach.
- Holding the strap with both hands, begin to pull your foot up toward your rear end.
- Relax and hold the stretch, ensuring proper breathing.

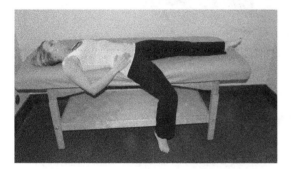

- Lie on your back on the edge of your bed or table.
- Hang one leg off the side of the table.
- Relax and hold the stretch, ensuring proper breathing.

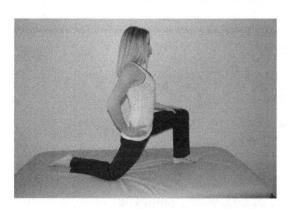

- Get down on both knees and place one foot forward in a lunge position.
- Take your weight down and forward, keeping your posture nice and tall.
- Relax and hold the stretch, ensuring proper breathing.

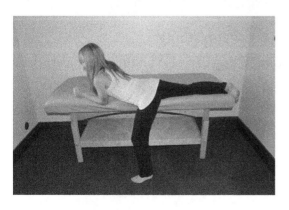

- Using your bed or table, lie on your stomach on the side of the table with one leg supporting you on the ground.
- Put your elbows underneath your shoulders and rise up, looking straight ahead. Focus on pushing your thigh into the table.
- Relax and hold the position, ensuring proper breathing.

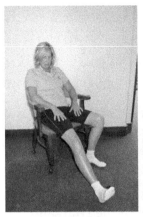 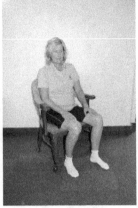

- Sitting in a chair, start with your leg straightened.
- Keeping your posture tall, slowly move your heel in under the chair.
- Relax and hold the stretch, ensuring proper breathing.

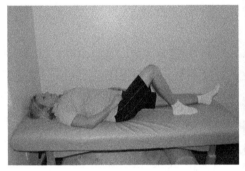 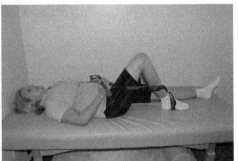

- Lie on the floor/bed with both legs in a straightened position.
- Keeping your foot touching the floor or bed, slowly bend your knee, bringing your heel in toward your glutes.
- Relax and hold the stretch, ensuring proper breathing.
- As you get more movement in your knee, you can also begin to use a strap or towel to help pull your foot back.

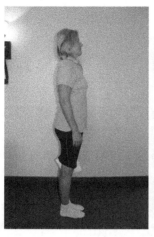 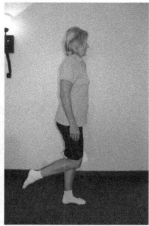

- In a standing position, place a towel between your knees.
- Squeezing the towel, slowly bend your knee, bringing your foot up behind you.
- Don't let the towel fall.
- Relax and hold the stretch, ensuring proper breathing.
- Hold on to the wall or other stationary object for stability. **(Intermediate)**

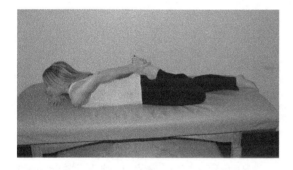

- Lie flat on your stomach.
- Pull your leg up toward your rear end and grab your ankle.
- Pull your foot in toward your rear end.
- Relax and hold the stretch, ensuring proper breathing. **(Intermediate)**

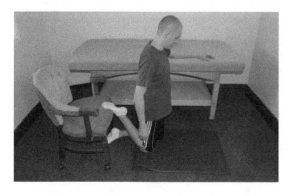

- Holding onto a stable surface, kneel on the ground.
- Lift your foot and place it on top of a chair.
- Keep your posture nice and tall, even with a slightly arched back.
- Relax and hold the stretch, ensuring proper breathing. **(Intermediate)**

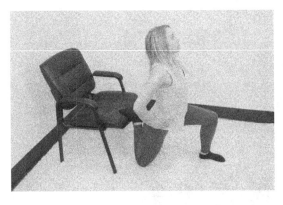

- Holding onto a stable surface, kneel on the ground.
- Lift your foot and place it on top of a chair.
- Move your other leg forward into a lunge position.
- Take your weight down and forward, keeping your posture nice and tall.
- Relax and hold the stretch, ensuring proper breathing. **(Intermediate)**

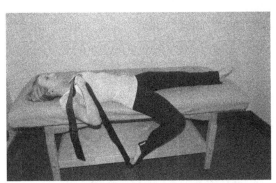

- Place a T-Stretch strap around your foot. Keep a hold of the strap.
- Lie on your back on the edge of your bed or table.
- Hang your leg off the side of the table and pull your foot up.
- Relax and hold the stretch, ensuring proper breathing. **(Intermediate)**

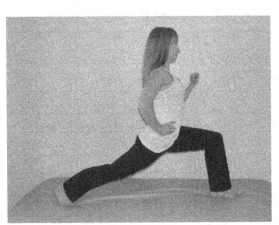

- Standing with your feet together, place one leg forward into a lunge position.
- Keeping your back leg straight and your forward knee above your heel, move your weight down toward the ground. Ensure your posture is nice and tall.
- Relax and hold the position, ensuring proper breathing. **(Intermediate)**

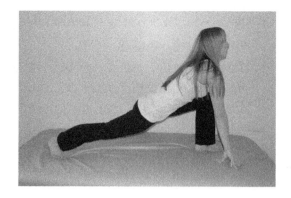

- Standing with your feet together, place one leg forward into a lunge position.
- Keeping your back leg straight and your forward knee above your heel, lean forward at the hips and place both hands on the ground.
- Move your weight down toward the ground.
- Relax and hold the position, ensuring proper breathing. **(Intermediate)**

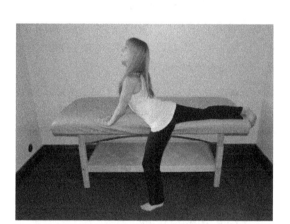

- Using your bed or table, lie on your stomach on the side of the table with one leg supporting you on the ground.
- Place your hands underneath your shoulders and rise up, looking straight ahead. Focus on pushing your thigh into the table.
- Relax and hold the position, ensuring proper breathing. **(Intermediate)**

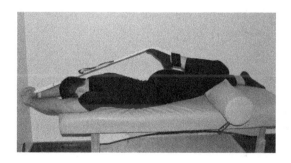

- Lying on your stomach, place a riser like a pillow or the foam roller just above your knee.
- Place the strap around your foot and pull your foot toward your head.
- Relax and hold the stretch, ensuring proper breathing. **(Intermediate)**

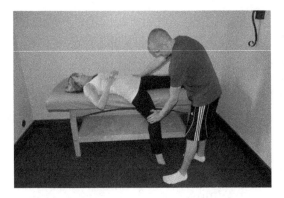

- Lie on your back on the side of a table with one leg hanging down.
- Have a partner assist you by holding down on the hip on the table and slowly pushing down on the knee of the hanging leg.
- Relax and hold the stretch, ensuring proper breathing. **(Intermediate)**

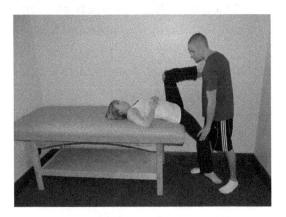

- Place your tailbone at the edge of the table and lie back.
- Your partner will place one foot at his/her chest while your other leg hangs down.
- Your partner pushes the knee down slowly until a stretch is felt.
- Relax and hold the stretch, ensuring proper breathing. **(Intermediate)**

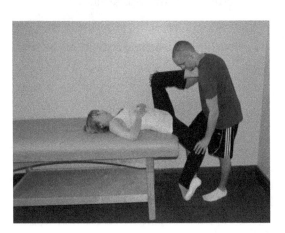

- Place your tail bone at the edge of the table and lie back.
- Your partner will place one foot at his/her chest while your other leg hangs down.
- Your partner pushes the knee down and uses his/her foot to slowly push your foot back toward the table.
- Relax and hold the stretch, ensuring proper breathing. **(Intermediate)**

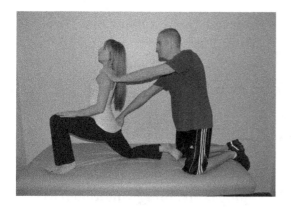

- Get down on both knees and place one foot out into a lunge position. Keeping your posture tall, move your body forward and hips down toward the floor.
- Have your partner place his/her fist just above your glutes and have them push down and forward.
- Relax and hold the stretch, ensuring proper breathing. **(Intermediate)**

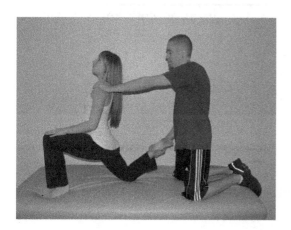

- Get down on both knees and place one foot out into a lunge position. Keeping your posture tall, move your body forward and hips down toward the floor.
- Have your partner grab the top of your foot and GENTLY pull your foot up off the ground.
- Relax and hold the stretch, ensuring proper breathing. **(Intermediate)**

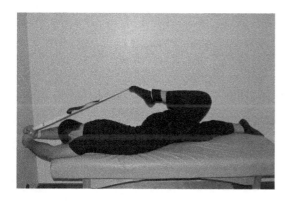

- Place a T-Stretch strap around your ankle and up over your toes.
- Lie on your stomach, holding the strap behind your head.
- Pull the strap over your head, lifting your knee off the ground.
- Relax and hold the stretch, ensuring proper breathing. **(Intermediate)**

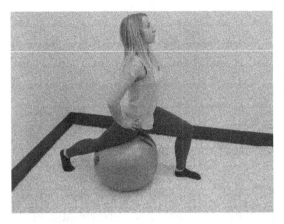

- Place one leg forward into a lunge position, straddling the ball.
- Keeping your back leg straight and your front knee above your heel, move your weight down toward the ground. Ensure your posture is nice and tall.
- Relax and hold the position, ensuring proper breathing. **(Intermediate)**

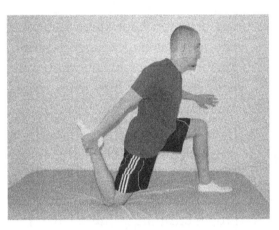

- Get down on both knees and place one foot forward in a lunge position.
- Reach behind you and take hold of your foot. Pull it up toward your hip. If needed, hold on to a stable object to help with balance.
- Take your weight down and forward, keeping your posture nice and tall.
- Relax and hold the stretch, ensuring proper breathing. **(Advanced)**

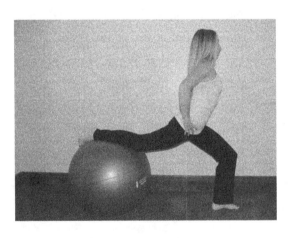

- Straddling the ball, place your shin and knee on top of the ball.
- Keeping your posture nice and tall, bend your front knee and lower your body toward the ground.
- Push your knee and shin into the ball as you lower your hip flexor down.
- Relax and hold the stretch, ensuring proper breathing. **(Advanced)**

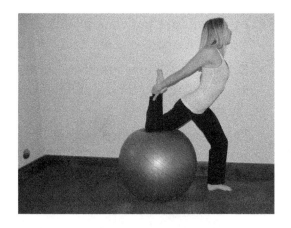

- Straddling the ball, place your shin and knee on top of the ball.
- Keeping your posture nice and tall, bend your front knee and lower your body toward the ground.
- Push your knee and shin into the ball as you lower your hip flexor down.
- Grab your foot and slowly pull your foot up toward your butt.
- Relax and hold the stretch, ensuring proper breathing. (**Advanced**)

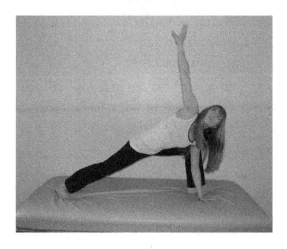

- Place your left leg forward into a lunge position.
- Keeping your right leg straight and your left knee above your heel, lean forward at the hips and place your left hand on the inside of your left foot.
- Pushing your left elbow into your knee, turn your body, and reach to the sky with your right arm.
- Relax and hold the position, ensuring proper breathing. (**Advanced**)

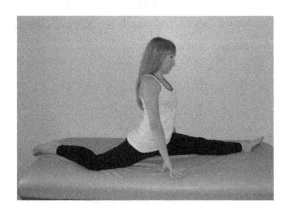

- Standing with your feet together, place one leg forward, and slowly begin to slide your feet further apart.
- Keeping your posture nice and tall, move down into a slide split position. Stabilize yourself with your hands if needed.
- Relax and hold the position, ensuring proper breathing. (**Advanced**)

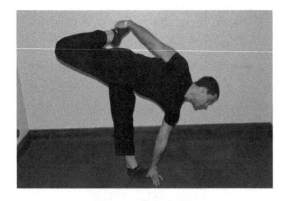

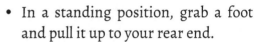

- In a standing position, grab a foot and pull it up to your rear end.
- Keeping hold of your foot, slowly lean forward and touch your hand to the floor.
- Keep your posture nice and tall.
- Relax and hold the position, ensuring proper breathing. **(Advanced)**

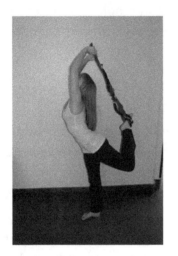

- Standing with both feet together, bring your foot up behind you and place a strap around your foot.
- Holding onto the strap, bring your hands above your head and pull up and in on your foot.
- With your posture nice and tall and a slight arch in your body, look up toward the ceiling.
- Relax and hold the stretch, ensuring proper breathing. **(Advanced)**

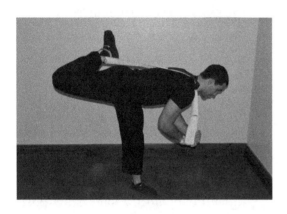

- Place the T-Stretch strap around your ankle and place the strap over your shoulder.
- Keeping your base leg straight, lean your body forward to a 90-degree angle from your leg as you pull your heel to your rear end.
- Relax and hold the stretch, ensuring proper breathing. **(Advanced)**

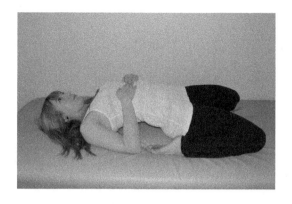

- Get down on both knees.
- Place your hands on the floor behind you and slowly lower your back to the ground.
- Relax and hold the stretch, ensuring proper breathing. **(Advanced)**
- This stretch can place a tremendous amount of pressure on the knees.

HIPS AND LOWER BACK

Unfortunately, mobility of the hip is a problem that most individuals will deal with at some point in their lives. When talking about the hip, I am referring to some of the most powerful muscles in the human body—a group of muscles that are responsible for running, jumping, and walking. I grouped the stretches for your hips and lower back together because they work hand in hand with each other. Some common problems with tight muscles in these two areas are:

- Arthritic pain
- Lower back pain
- Hamstring pain
- Sciatica (pain in your sciatic nerve that can be caused by a tight piriformis)
- Knee pain
- Poor balance
- Poor posture

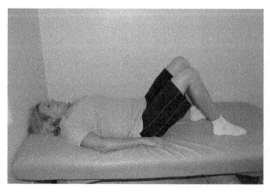

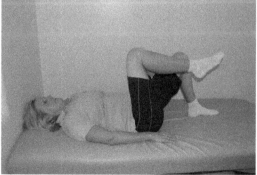

- Lying on your back, bend both of your knees.
- Keeping that same angle in your knee, raise your foot off the table.
- Try to press your lower back into the floor/bed (pelvic tilt) as you raise your foot.
- Relax and hold the stretch, ensuring proper breathing.

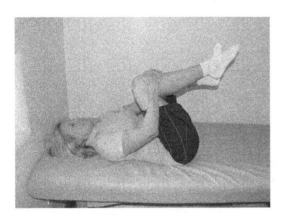

- Lie on your back.
- Pull your knees up to your chest.
- Grasp your knees with your hands or arms and slowly pull them into your chest.
- Relax and hold the stretch, ensuring proper breathing.
- Recommended after any type of rotational stretch.

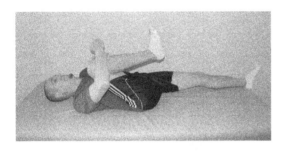

- Lie on your back.
- Pull one knee up toward your chest.
- Grasp your knee and pull it in slowly toward the chest.
- Relax and hold the stretch, ensuring proper breathing.

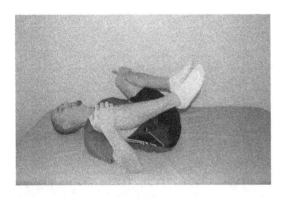

- Lie on your back.
- Pull both knees up toward your chest.
- Grasping your knees with your hands, pull your knees in toward your chest and out away from each other.
- Relax and hold the stretch, ensuring proper breathing.

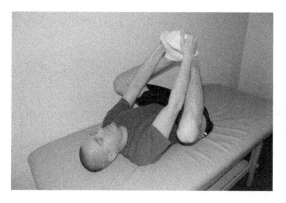

- Lie on your back.
- Pull both knees up toward your chest.
- Place the inside edges of your feet together.
- Grasp the outside of your feet and pull in toward your chest.
- Relax and hold the stretch, ensuring proper breathing.

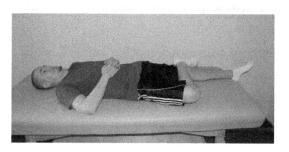

- Lie on your back.
- Place your right ankle on your left knee.
- Rest your knee down to the table.
- Relax and hold the stretch, ensuring proper breathing.

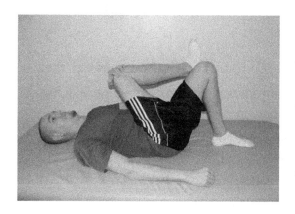

- Lie on your back with both knees bent.
- Place your right ankle on your left knee.
- Using your left hand, grasp your right knee and pull your knee down toward your chest.
- Relax and hold the stretch, ensuring proper breathing.

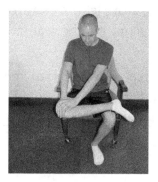

- In a seated position, place your right ankle on your left knee.
- Sitting in a nice and tall position, slowly push your knee down.
- Relax and hold the stretch, ensuring proper breathing.

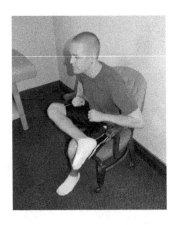

- In a seated position, place your right ankle on your left knee.
- Keeping your posture nice and tall, slowly lean forward at the hips.
- Relax and hold the stretch, ensuring proper breathing.

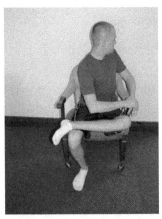

- In a seated position, place your left ankle on your right knee.
- Keeping your posture nice and tall, slowly rotate your upper body to the left.
- Relax and hold the stretch, ensuring proper breathing.

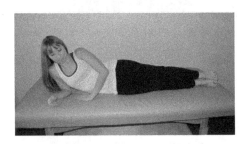

- Lie on your side with your legs together.
- Prop yourself up on your elbow, placing the elbow under your shoulder.
- Support yourself with your other arm.
- Relax and hold the stretch, ensuring proper breathing.

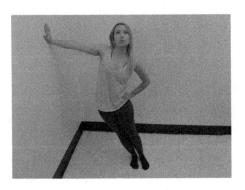

- Standing an arm's length away from a wall, place your hand on the wall at shoulder height.
- With your feet together, lean your hips in toward the wall.
- Relax and hold the stretch, ensuring proper breathing.

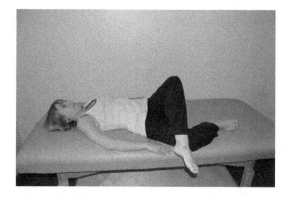

- Lie on your back, place your left ankle on your right knee.
- Pull your right foot in and lay the outside your right knee down on the floor.
- Continue to pull your right knee and foot in until you feel a stretch.
- Relax and hold the stretch, ensuring proper breathing.

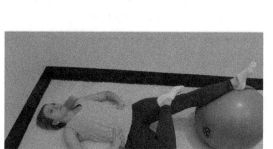

- Lying on your back, place your leg straight out on top of a therapy ball.
- Place your ankle just above your knee.
- Relax and hold the stretch, ensuring proper breathing.
- Repeat on the other side.

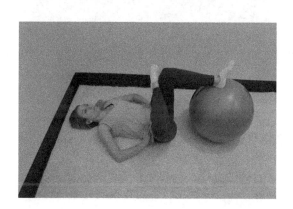

- Lying on your back, place your leg straight out on top of the ball.
- Place your ankle just above your knee.
- Slowly bend your knee and pull the ball in toward your body until you feel a stretch.
- Relax and hold the stretch, ensuring proper breathing.

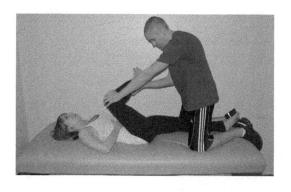

- Lying on your back, have your partner take hold of your leg, placing one hand on the side of your knee and the other hand on your ankle.
- Keeping your leg at a 90-degree angle, have your partner GENTLY push your knee toward your chest.

- Relax and hold the stretch, ensuring proper breathing.
- Communicate with your partner, letting him/her know when you feel the stretch.

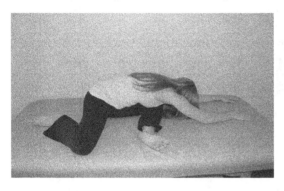

- In a seated position, bend one leg and place it behind you and bend your forward leg to a 90-degree angle.
- Keeping your posture nice and tall, lean forward toward your knee.
- Relax and hold the stretch, ensuring proper breathing. **(Intermediate)**

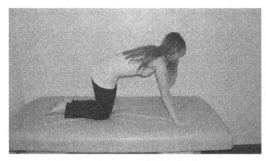 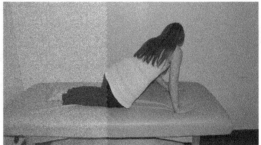

- Begin this stretch on your hands and knees.
- Rotate your hips and lower them toward the floor.
- Relax and hold the stretch, ensuring proper breathing. **(Intermediate)**

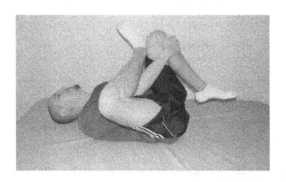

- Lie on your back with both knees bent.
- Place your right ankle on your left knee.

- Take your right arm through your legs and grasp your knee. Take your left hand and place it on your right hand, interlocking your fingers.
- Pull your left knee toward your chest, feeling this stretch in your right hip.
- Relax and hold the stretch, ensuring proper breathing. **(Intermediate)**

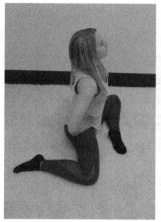 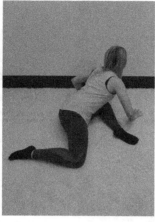 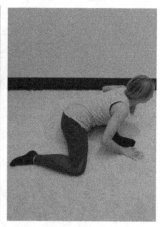

- From a seated position, bend your knee with your foot behind you.
- Bend your opposite leg in front of you and place your foot against the other knee.
- Keeping your posture tall, bend forward at your hips.
- Relax and hold the stretch, ensuring proper breathing.
- This is a great stretch because you can lean forward in different directions and stretch different muscles in the hip. **(Intermediate)**

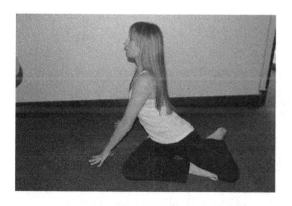

- From a seated position, bend one knee and place it behind you.
- Bend your opposite knee and place your foot against your leg.
- Keeping your posture tall, rotate your body toward your front leg.
- Lean into your leg and place both hands on the floor.
- Relax and hold the stretch, ensuring proper breathing. **(Intermediate)**

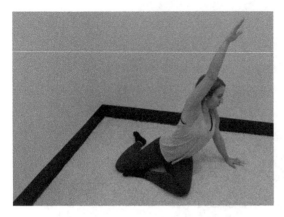

- From a seated position, bend one knee and place it behind you. Bend your opposite knee and place your foot against your leg.
- Keeping your posture tall, rotate your body toward your front leg and place your back hand on the floor.
- Keeping your chest up, reach your forward arm over your head, extending your arm.
- Relax and hold the stretch, ensuring proper breathing. **(Intermediate)**

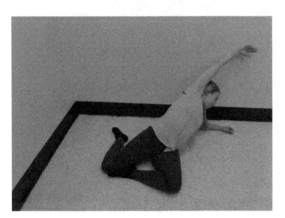

- From a seated position, bend one knee and place it behind you. Bend your opposite knee and place your foot against your leg.
- Keeping your posture tall, rotate your body toward your front leg and place your back elbow on the floor.
- Keeping your chest up, reach your forward arm over your head, extending your arm.
- Relax and hold the stretch, ensuring proper breathing. **(Intermediate)**

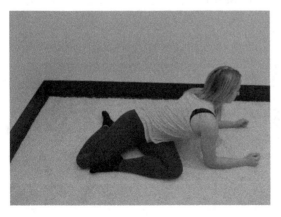

- From a seated position, bend one knee and place it behind you. Bend your opposite knee and place your foot against your leg.
- Keeping your posture tall, rotate your body toward your front leg and place both elbows on the floor.
- Keep your posture nice and tall.
- Relax and hold the stretch, ensuring proper breathing. **(Intermediate)**

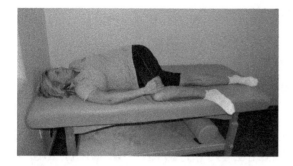

- Lie on your side, bend your top leg and place it at a 90-degree angle.
- Slowly push your top shoulder back to the ground, holding your upper knee down to the floor.
- Relax and hold the stretch, ensuring proper breathing. **(Intermediate)**

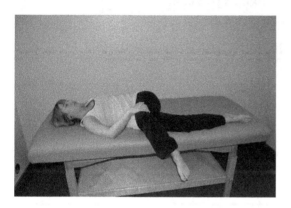

- Lie on your side (close to the edge of a bed or table), bend your top leg to a 90-degree angle so the top leg hangs off the table.
- Slowly push your top shoulder back to the bed or table while holding your upper knee down.
- Relax and hold the stretch, ensuring proper breathing. **(Intermediate)**

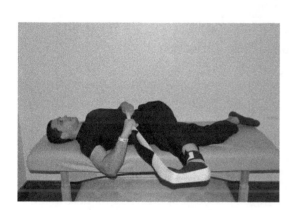

- Place a T-Stretch strap around your left foot and lie on your right side.
- Holding the strap, keep your left leg straight.
- Slowly push your left shoulder back on the floor/bed and pull your left leg up toward your head.
- Relax and hold the stretch, ensuring proper breathing. **(Intermediate)**

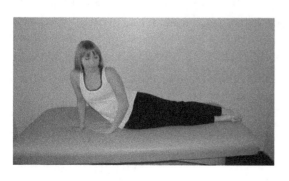

- Lie on your side with your legs together.
- Prop yourself up on your hand, placing your hand under your shoulder.
- Support yourself with your other arm.
- Relax and hold the stretch, ensuring proper breathing. **(Intermediate)**

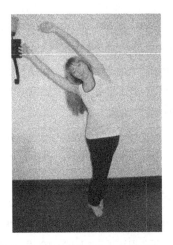

- Stand with your feet together and your posture nice and tall.
- Cross one leg in front of the other.
- Raise your arms high above your head and lean to the side where your foot is crossed.
- Keep your posture nice and tall and pointed forward. Try not to turn your body. Reach as high as you can.
- Relax and hold the stretch, ensuring proper breathing. **(Intermediate)**

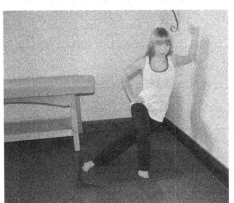

- Stand approximately elbow length away from the wall.
- Take the leg closest to the wall and cross it behind you. Slide it away from the wall as you slowly lower down toward the ground. Do not let your forward knee get past your toes.
- Relax and hold the stretch, ensuring proper breathing. **(Advanced)**

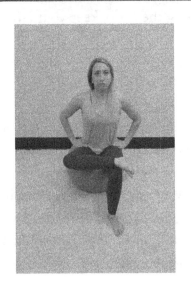

- Sitting on a therapy ball, place your ankle on your knee.
- Keep your posture nice and tall, focusing on balance.
- Let your knee relax down toward the ground.
- Relax and hold the stretch, ensuring proper breathing. **(Advanced)**

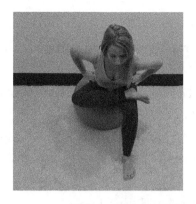

- Sitting on a therapy ball, place your ankle on your knee.
- Keeping your posture nice and tall, lean forward. Focus on your balance.
- Relax and hold the stretch, ensuring proper breathing. **(Advanced)**

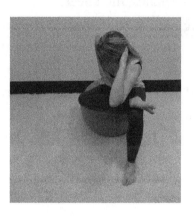

- Sitting on a therapy ball, place your ankle on your knee.
- Place the opposite hand on the back of your head. Keeping your posture nice and tall, rotate your elbow down toward your knee.
- Focus on your balance.
- Relax and hold the stretch, ensuring proper balance. **(Advanced)**

LOWER BACK AND ABS

I am sure you have heard that exercising and making our abdominals strong will help ease lower back pain, which is true; however, *tight* abdominal muscles can also cause some serious problems. When these muscles are ignored and get tight, they can actually place pressure on the organs in our body, forcing them to move up in our thoracic cavity. I, unfortunately, have dealt with this issue myself. It actually started affecting my breathing and gave me tremendous abdominal pain. Now, many of these stretches have become my favorites. Other problems that can arise are:

- Lower back pain
- Mid-/upper back pain
- Poor digestion
- Cramping
- Chest pain
- Menstrual pain
- Hernias

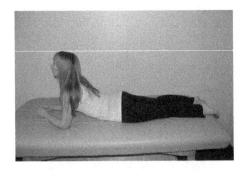

- Lie on your stomach.
- Place your elbows underneath your shoulders and rise up. Look straight ahead.
- Relax and hold the stretch, ensuring proper breathing.
- Be warned, this stretch can place strain on the lower back.

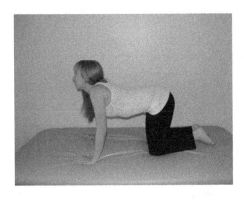

- Get on your hands and knees.
- Breathing out, let your chest and stomach sink down to the ground as you raise your head up.
- Relax and hold the stretch, ensuring proper breathing.
- Combine this stretch with the stretch below for a great functional movement for the spine.

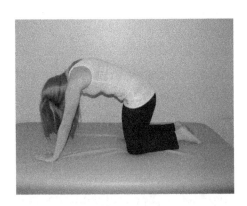

- Get on your hands and knees.
- Breathing in, arch your back as high as it will comfortably allow. Lower your head down toward the floor.
- Relax and hold the stretch, ensuring proper breathing.
- Combine this stretch with the stretch above for a great functional movement for the spine.

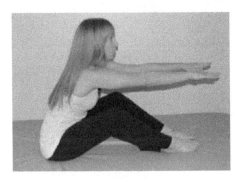

- In a seated position, slightly bend both knees.
- Keeping your posture nice and tall, slowly reach forward.

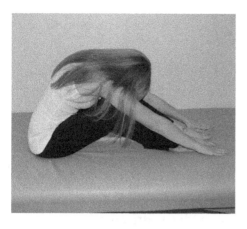

- Relax and hold the stretch, ensuring proper breathing.
- In a seated position, slightly bend both knees.
- Keeping your posture tall, slowly reach forward.
- Lower your arms, letting your head sink down between your knees. Slide your hands even further forward if you are able.
- Relax and hold the stretch, ensuring proper breathing.

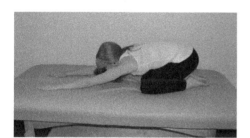

- Position yourself on your hands and knees.
- Sit back into your heels and push your chest down to the floor. Ensure your arms are reaching out over your head.
- Relax and hold the stretch, ensuring proper breathing.

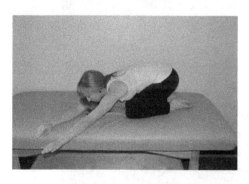

- Position yourself on your hands and knees.
- Sit back into your heels and push your chest down to the floor. Ensure your arms are reaching out over your head.
- Slowly reach both arms to the side.
- Relax and hold the stretch, ensuring proper breathing.

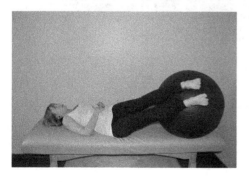

- Lying on your back, place your feet on top of a therapy ball.
- Use your feet to turn the ball to the side, rotating your legs to the side as well.
- Relax and hold the stretch, ensuring proper breathing.
- For traction, do this with shoes or bare feet.

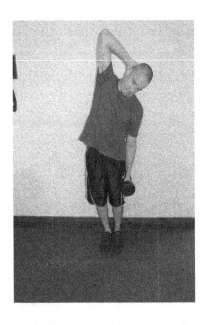

- Standing up, place one hand behind your head.
- Holding a weight in your other hand, bend to the side. Keep your posture nice and tall and ensure the hand holding the weight stays up against your body and slides down the side of your leg. Don't bend forward.
- Feet can be together or, if you need more balance, shoulder-width apart.
- Relax and hold the stretch, ensuring proper breathing.

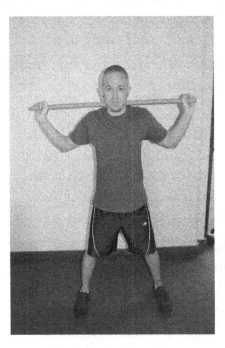
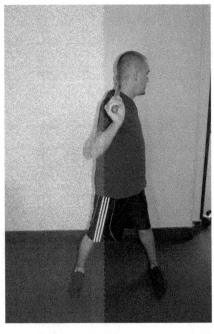

- Stand with your feet approximately shoulder-width apart.
- Carefully place and hold a pole of some sort on your upper back and shoulders.
- Keeping your posture nice and tall, rotate your upper body to the side.
- Relax and hold the stretch, ensuring proper breathing.

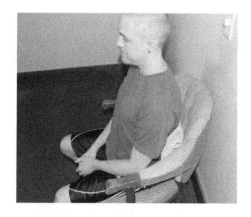

- Sitting in a chair, roll up a bath towel and place it at various positions along your back.
- Keep your posture nice and tall while sitting normally. Don't push your back into the towel.
- Relax and hold the stretch, ensuring proper breathing.

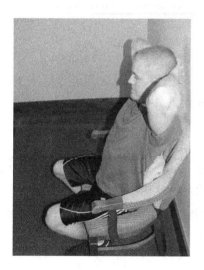

- Sitting in a chair, roll up a bath towel and place it at your mid-back.
- Place your hands on the back of your head.
- Keeping your posture nice and tall, slowly arch back into the towel.
- Relax and hold the stretch, ensuring proper breathing.

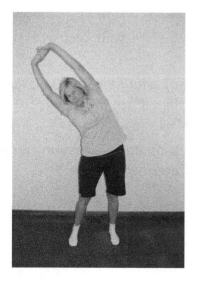

- Stand with your feet approximately shoulder-width apart.
- Interlock your fingers and raise your arms over your head.
- Keeping your posture nice and tall, lean to the side and focus on pushing the palms of your hands up and out away from your body.
- Relax and hold the stretch, ensuring proper breathing.

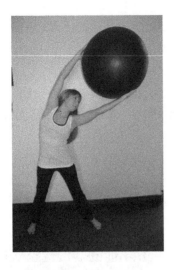

- Stand with your feet approximately shoulder-width apart.
- Holding on to a therapy ball, extend your arms over your head.
- Keeping your posture nice and tall, lean to the side and focus on pushing the ball up and away from your body.
- Relax and hold the stretch, ensuring proper breathing.

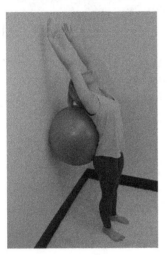

- Place a therapy ball against the wall.
- Position the ball so that you are resting your lower to mid-back against the ball.
- With your hands stretched up above your head or hands behind your head, lean back against the ball. I tell my clients to try to take the shape of the ball.
- Relax and hold the stretch, ensuring proper breathing.

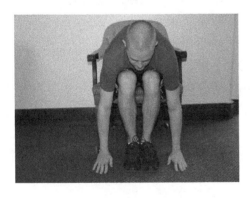

- Sit in a chair with your feet and knees together.
- Keeping your posture nice and tall, slowly lower to the floor. Place your hands on each side of your feet.
- Relax and hold the stretch, ensuring proper breathing. **(Intermediate)**

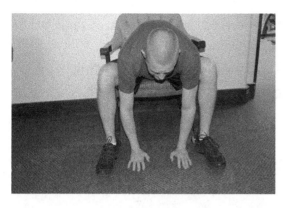

- Sit in a chair with your feet and knees wider than shoulder-width.
- Keeping your posture nice and tall, slowly lower to the floor in between your knees and feet.
- Relax and hold the stretch, ensuring proper breathing. **(Intermediate)**

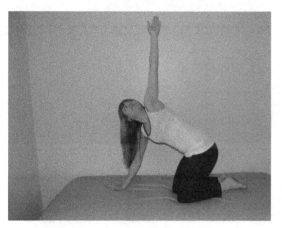

- Get on your hands and knees.
- Take one arm and rotate your body. Reach as high as you can. Look in the direction of your arm.
- Relax and hold the stretch, ensuring proper breathing. **(Intermediate)**

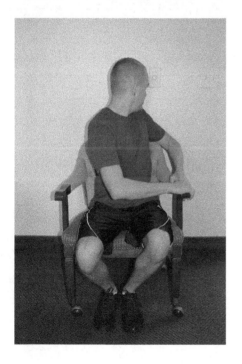

- Sit in a chair or on the end of your bed.
- Keeping your posture tall, rotate your body to the side. You can use the arm of the chair or the cushion to help you rotate a little more.
- Relax and hold the position, ensuring proper breathing. **(Intermediate)**

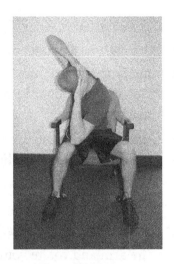

- In a seated position, place your hands behind your head.
- Spread your legs shoulder-width apart.
- Rotate and take your left elbow to your right knee.
- Relax and hold each position, ensuring proper breathing. **(Intermediate)**

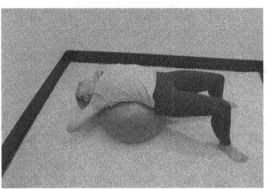

- Begin by sitting on a therapy ball. Slowly roll yourself down into a lying position.
- Position yourself so that your mid-back is centered on the ball. Keep your knees bent for better support.
- Extend your arms over your head or place them behind your head and slowly relax your body to take the shape of the ball.
- Relax and hold the stretch, ensuring proper breathing. **(Intermediate)**

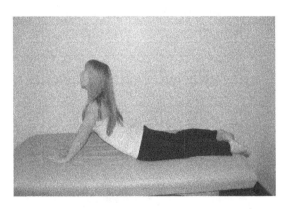

- Lie on your stomach.
- Place your hands underneath your shoulders and rise up. Look straight ahead.
- Relax and hold the stretch, ensuring proper breathing.
- This stretch can place a tremendous amount of stress on the lower back. **(Intermediate)**

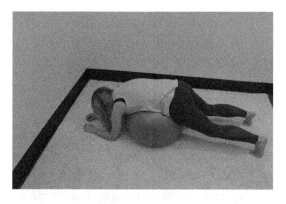

- Lie with your stomach on a therapy ball.
- Let your body sink down and take the shape of the ball. You can also place your feet against the wall for more stability.
- Relax and hold the stretch, ensuring proper breathing. **(Intermediate)**

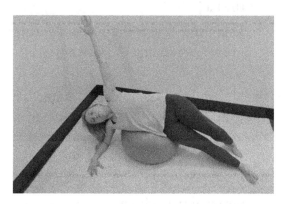

- Lay your side on a therapy ball with your hand and feet on the floor for stability.
- Stretch your upper arm out above your head.
- Slowly lower your upper body, taking the shape of the ball.
- Relax and hold the stretch, ensuring proper breathing. **(Intermediate)**

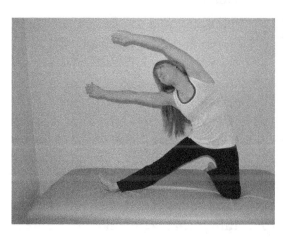

- Begin this position on your knees.
- Straighten one leg and place it out to the side with your toes pointed up.
- Raise your hands above your head and bend to the side of the straightened leg.
- Keep your posture nice and tall and reach as far as you can.
- Relax and hold the stretch, ensuring proper breathing. **(Intermediate)**

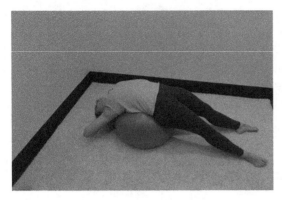

- Begin by sitting on a therapy ball. Slowly roll yourself down into a lying position.
- Position yourself so that your mid-back is centered on the ball.
- Keeping your legs straight, extend your arms over your head or place them behind your head and slowly relax your body to take the shape of the ball.
- Relax and hold the stretch, ensuring proper breathing. **(Advanced)**

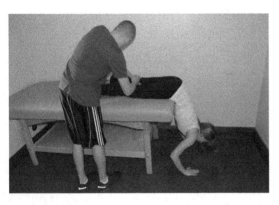

- Lie on your stomach, situated so your body hangs off the side of a table/bed, bending you at your waist.
- Have your partner tightly hold your legs down while you slightly support yourself with your hands on the floor.
- Relax and hold the stretch, ensuring proper breathing. **(Advanced)**

UPPER BACK

Most of our daily activities are responsible for the aches and pains we feel throughout the week. Whether your job is sitting at a desk behind a computer or a dentist having to position yourself to look in someone's mouth, our actions cause consequences in our bodies. Due to these daily actions, we tend to develop poor posture, which can lead to upper back pain and discomfort. Tightness in these muscles can make it very difficult to do things that we all take for granted, like raising our hands above our head or even moving our neck. Other issues that may arise are:

- Arthritic pain
- Neck pain

- Shoulder impingement
- Bursitis (inflammation of a bursa, which is a fluid-filled sac that decreases friction in your joints)
- Tingling in your arms
- Frozen shoulder

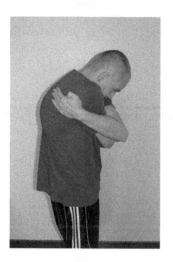

- In a standing or seated position, cross your arms and give yourself a big hug.
- Round your shoulders forward and lower your head to your chest while you pull forward on your back with your hands.
- Relax and hold the stretch, ensuring proper breathing.

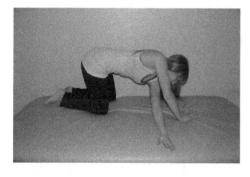

- Start this stretch from your hands and knees.
- Keeping one arm straight, slide your other arm under your body and lower your shoulder to the ground. Reach with the arm on the floor.
- Relax and hold the stretch, ensuring proper breathing.
- Placing your palm down will intensify the stretch.

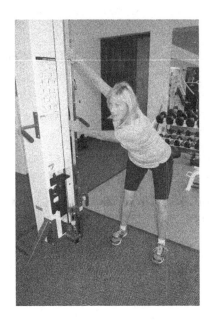

- Begin by standing with your side approximately one foot away from a door jamb or a secure post.
- With your feet shoulder-width apart, grasp a door jamb or secure post with both hands (thumbs should point toward each other).
- Place the closest hand on the top about head height and the lower hand even with the lower portion of your chest.
- Making sure your hips are pointed forward, pull with your lower arm, and push with your upper arm.
- Relax and hold the stretch, ensuring proper breathing.

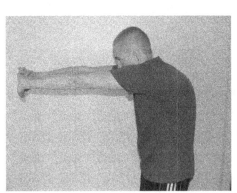

- In a standing or seated position, interlock your fingers.
- Extend your arms straight out in front of you with your palms facing out.
- Let your shoulders round forward.
- Relax and hold the stretch, ensuring proper breathing.

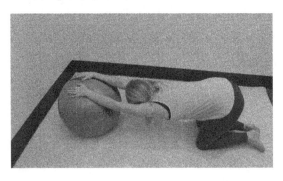

- While on your knees, place your arms straight out with your palms down on a therapy ball.
- Keeping your arms straight, slowly lower your chest to the ground.
- Relax and hold the stretch, ensuring proper breathing.

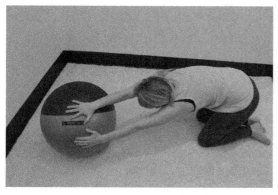

- While on your knees, place your arms straight out with your palms down on a therapy ball.
- With your arms straight, slowly lower your chest to the ground and rotate the ball to the side.
- Relax and hold the stretch, ensuring proper breathing. Repeat on the other side.

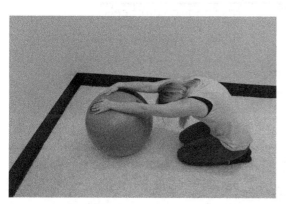

- While on your knees, place your arms straight out with your palms down on a therapy ball.
- With your arms straight, slowly rise up, rounding your upper back and lowering your head.
- Reach your arms out as far as you can.
- Relax and hold the stretch, ensuring proper breathing.

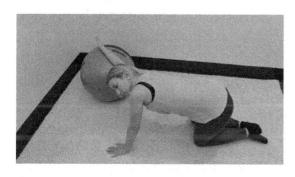

- While on your knees, place your right arm slightly out on an angle with your thumb up.
- Slowly lower your right shoulder down toward the ground.
- Relax and hold the stretch, ensuring proper breathing.

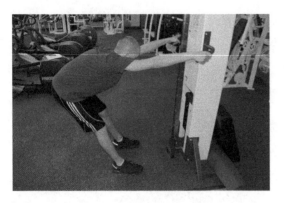

- Take hold of a secure object. Stand close enough that your arms have a slight bend.
- Slowly move your chest toward the ground while pushing your rear end back.
- Relax and hold the stretch, ensuring proper breathing.

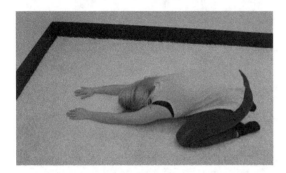

- On your hands and knees, lower your rear end to your heels.
- Reach your hands out above your head and push your chest to the floor.
- Relax and hold the stretch, ensuring proper breathing.

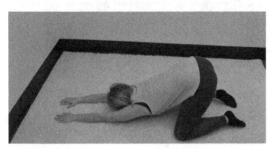

- On your hands and knees, slide your hands slightly in front of your head.
- Slowly move your chest down toward the ground, keeping your hips up.
- Relax and hold the stretch, ensuring proper breathing.

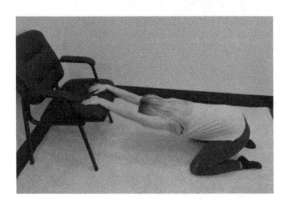

- From your knees, place your hands and forearms on the seat of a chair.
- Slowly move your chest down toward the ground keeping your hips up.
- Relax and hold the stretch, ensuring proper breathing.

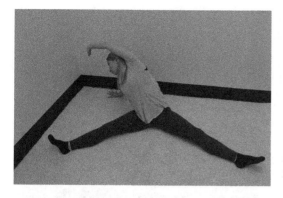

- From a seated position on the floor, spread your legs and place your hand on the floor to the side and behind you.
- Leaning on your hand, reach the other arm up over your head.
- Relax and hold the stretch, ensuring proper breathing.

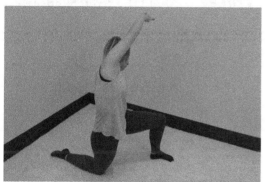

- From a kneeling position, bend one leg and place your foot out to the side.
- Reach your opposite side arm up and over your head and slowly lean toward your knee.
- Relax and hold the stretch, ensuring proper breathing.

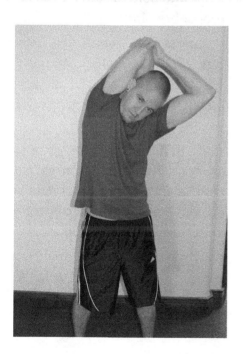

- Keep your posture nice and tall from either a standing or sitting position.
- Pull your elbow over your head.
- Grab your elbow and pull back. Slowly lean your upper body to the side.
- Relax and hold the stretch, ensuring proper breathing.

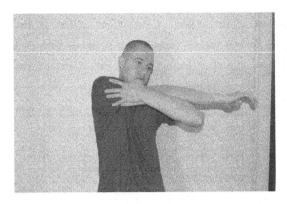

- Keep your posture nice and tall from either a standing or sitting position.
- Reach across your body with your arm.
- With the other hand, grab the back of your arm.
- Pull your arm slightly out toward the other side of your body.
- Relax and hold the stretch, ensuring proper breathing.

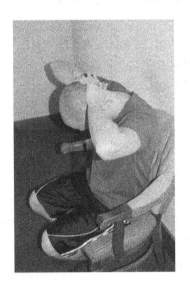

- Keep your posture nice and tall from either a standing or sitting position.
- Interlock your fingers and place them on the back of your head.
- Slowly pull your head down.
- Relax and hold the stretch, ensuring proper breathing.
- If you slowly move your elbows forward and slightly round your shoulders, you will feel the stretch moving down from your neck into your upper back.

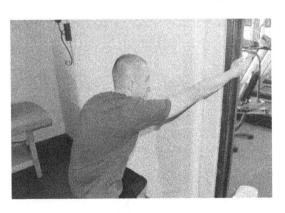

- With one hand, hold on to a door jamb or a pole. The pole or door jamb should be straight in front of you. Your thumb should be on top.
- Slowly lower your body down (squat down) and away from your hand.
- Relax and hold the stretch, ensuring proper breathing. **(Intermediate)**

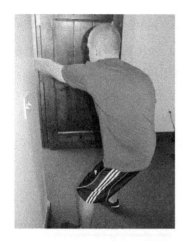

- Stand with a pole or door jamb off-center.
- With the arm furthest away, reach across your body and grab hold of the pole. Your thumb should be on the bottom.
- Slowly lower your body down into a squat position.
- Relax and hold the stretch, ensuring proper breathing. **(Intermediate)**

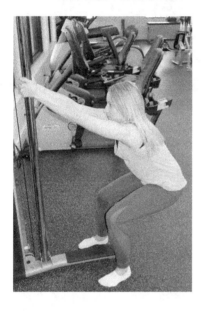

- Stand in front of a pole with your feet shoulder-width apart.
- Grab a secure post approximately at chest level. Stand just close enough to have your arms slightly bent.
- Keeping a firm hold on the pole, squat down, keeping your knees above your heels.
- Slightly leaning back and looking down toward the ground will intensify the stretch.
- Relax and hold the stretch, ensuring proper breathing. **(Intermediate)**

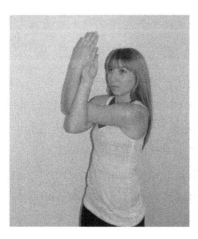

- Stand or sit, keeping your posture nice and tall.
- Reach your arms straight out in front of you, crossing them at your elbows.
- Bend both arms and place the palms of your hands together.
- Relax and hold the stretch, ensuring proper breathing. **(Intermediate)**

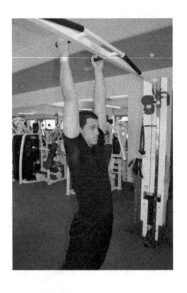

- Hold onto a bar overhead.
- Move your feet forward so your arms are slightly behind you.
- Place your weight on your heels and lean back into the stretch.
- Relax and hold the stretch, ensuring proper breathing. **(Intermediate)**

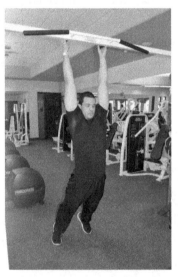

- Hold onto a bar overhead.
- Move your feet backward so your arms are reaching forward.
- Place your weight on your toes and lean forward into the stretch.
- Relax and hold the stretch, ensuring proper breathing. **(Intermediate)**

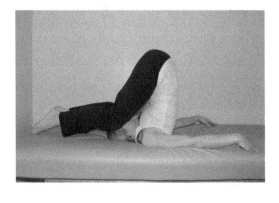

- Lie on your back.
- Bring your feet up and over your head, resting them on the floor.
- Keep your arms on the floor to give yourself more balance.
- Relax and hold the stretch, ensuring proper breathing. **(Advanced)**

HANDS AND FOREARMS

Tightness in the hands and forearms typically occurs from overuse of these muscles. Activities such as typing, sewing, and golfing can create tightness of these muscles. These symptoms definitely need to be treated; however, keep in mind that many problems can also be associated with tightness in your shoulders, neck, chest, and even in the upper back. Problems often associated with tightness in your hands and forearms are:

- Arthritic pain
- Carpal tunnel
- Hand weakness
- Golfer's elbow
- Tingling
- Pain

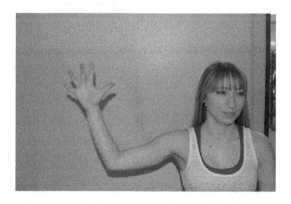

- Open your hands and spread your fingers as far apart from each other as you can.
- Relax and hold the stretch, ensuring proper breathing.

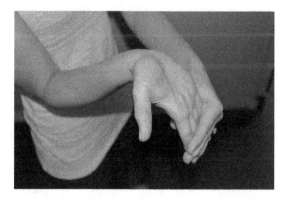

- Keeping your elbow bent and palm up, open your hand and keep your fingers together.
- Use your other hand to slowly pull back on your fingers.
- Relax and hold the stretch, ensuring proper breathing.

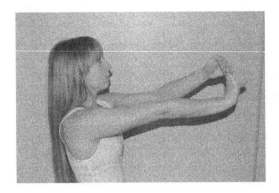

- Keeping your arm straight out in front of you, open your hand and keep your fingers together and pointing upward.
- Use your other hand to slowly pull back on your fingers.
- Relax and hold the stretch, ensuring proper breathing.

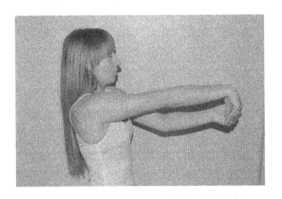

- Keeping your arm straight out in front of you, open your hand and keep your fingers together and pointing downward.
- Use your other hand to slowly pull back on the back of your hand.
- Relax and hold the stretch, ensuring proper breathing.

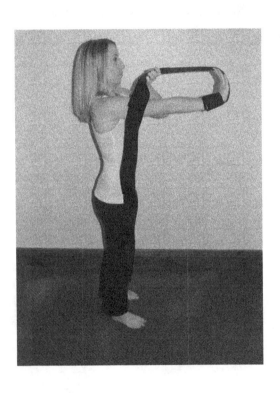

- Place the T-Stretch strap around your wrist. Extend the strap down the palm of your hand and over your fingertips.
- Using your other hand, gently pull the strap toward you. This will pull your fingers in toward your body.
- Use caution when doing this stretch. It can place pressure on your elbow, wrist, and fingers.
- Relax and hold the stretch, ensuring proper breathing.

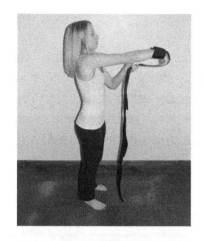

- Place the strap around your wrist, extending the strap over the back of your hand and over your fingertips.
- Using your other hand, gently pull the strap toward you. This again will pull your fingers in toward your body and stretch your upper forearm.
- Relax and hold the stretch, ensuring proper breathing.

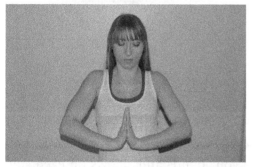

- Place the palms of your hands together.
- Slowly raise your elbows, keeping your palms together.
- Relax and hold the stretch, ensuring proper breathing. **(Intermediate)**

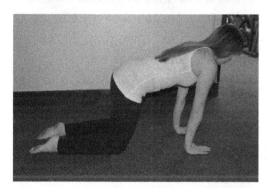

- Get on your hands and knees.
- Place your hands flat on the floor with your fingers pointed forward.
- Keeping the palms of your hands down on the floor, slowly move your body forward.
- Relax and hold the stretch, ensuring proper breathing. **(Intermediate)**

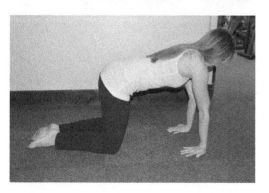

- Get on your hands and knees.
- Place your hands flat on the floor with your fingers pointed backward.
- Keeping the palms of your hands down on the floor, slowly move your body backward.
- Relax and hold the stretch, ensuring proper breathing. **(Advanced)**

ARMS, SHOULDER, AND CHEST

Our daily activities play such an enormous role in our posture and, of course, our overall flexibility. The muscles in our arms, shoulders, and chest are all connected and, typically, if one area is tight, so are the others. In order to relieve pain and tightness in one area, you need to stretch the other muscle groups as well. Tightness in this area can create chest pain and tingling in the hands, as well as:

- Shoulder impingement
- Frozen shoulder
- Bursitis and tendonitis
- Golfer's elbow
- Arthritic pain
- Poor posture

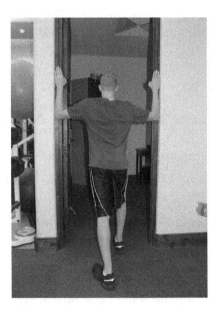

- Start by standing in a doorway. Bend your elbows to a 90-degree angle.
- Place your hands and elbows on each side of the doorway. I try to keep my elbows up at shoulder height. Changing the height will change the angle of the stretch.
- Place one leg forward through the doorway.
- Keeping your posture nice and tall, slowly lean your body forward into the stretch.
- Relax and hold the stretch, ensuring proper breathing.

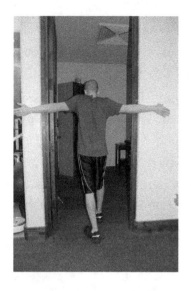

- Start by standing in a doorway. Straighten your arms and place them on each side of the doorway, approximately at shoulder height. Moving your hands up or down the doorway will change the angle of the stretch, so don't be afraid to experiment with your arm angle to feel what works best for you.
- Place one leg forward through the doorway.
- Keeping your posture nice and tall, slowly lean your body forward into the stretch.
- Relax and hold the stretch, ensuring proper breathing.

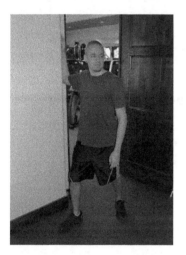

- In a standing position, place your arm against a doorway or other stable column.
- Place the leg of the side you are stretching forward.
- Keeping your elbow up at your shoulder height and your posture nice and tall, slowly lean forward and turn your body the opposite direction.
- Relax and hold the stretch, ensuring proper breathing.
- Turning your head the other direction will help to slightly intensify the stretch and you will add another great stretch for your neck.

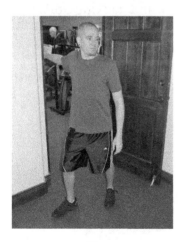

- In a standing position, place your hand against a doorway or other stable column.
- Place the leg of the side you are stretching forward.
- Keeping your hand above shoulder height and your posture nice and tall, slowly lean forward and turn your body the opposite direction.
- Relax and hold the stretch, ensuring proper breathing.
- This is a great stretch for your chest but can also stretch down the bicep and into the forearm.

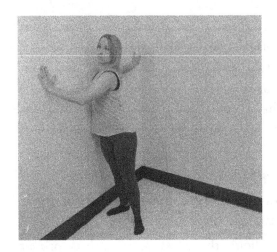

- Face a wall in a standing position.
- Place your hand, elbow, and shoulder against the wall.
- Move the opposite foot slightly away from the wall, and place your opposite palm on the wall.
- Keeping your hand, elbow, and shoulder against the wall, slowly turn your opposite shoulder away from the wall.
- Relax and hold the stretch, ensuring proper breathing.

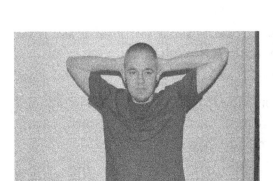

- In a standing or seated position, place both hands behind your head.
- Keeping your posture tall, slowly push your elbows back.
- Relax and hold the stretch, ensuring proper breathing.

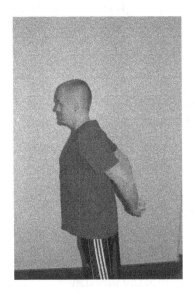

- In a standing position, take hold of your hands behind your back.
- Keeping your posture tall and looking forward, slowly push your hands back, away from your body. Think of pushing your chest out.
- Relax and hold the stretch, ensuring proper breathing.

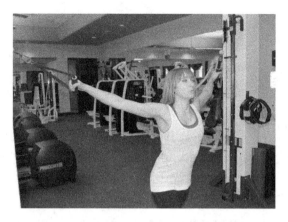

- Using a cable crossover machine, place both pullies above head height.
- Take both handles and move slightly forward until you feel tension.
- Keeping your posture tall, lean your body forward, sticking your chest out.
- Relax and hold the stretch, ensuring proper breathing.

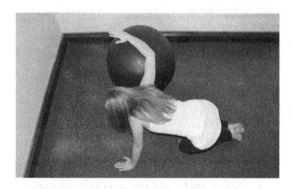

- From your hands and knees, place your elbow on a therapy ball, keeping your arm at a 90-degree angle.
- Slowly lower the same shoulder down toward the ground.
- Relax and hold the stretch, ensuring proper breathing.

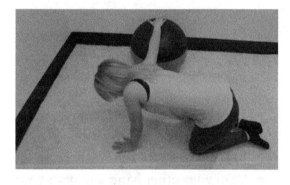

- From your hands and knees, place your straightened arm on a therapy ball.
- Slowly lower the same shoulder down toward the ground.
- Relax and hold the stretch, ensuring proper breathing.

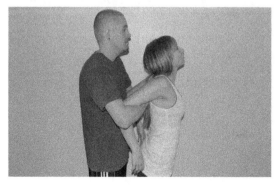

- In a standing position, have your partner hold underneath your bent arms with their hands on your back.
- Keeping your posture nice and tall, have your partner slowly squeeze your arms together.
- Relax and hold the stretch, ensuring proper breathing.

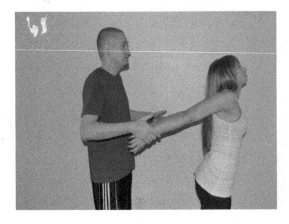

- In a standing position, have your partner hold your wrists with your arms straight behind you.
- Keeping your posture nice and tall, have your partner slowly raise and squeeze your arms together.
- Relax and hold the stretch, ensuring proper breathing.
- Communicate with your partner, letting him/ her know when you are feeling the stretch.

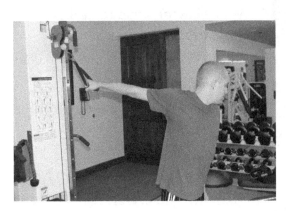

- Grab onto a fixed object behind you that is approximately shoulder height.
- Keeping your posture nice and tall, slowly move forward, stretching your arm behind you.
- Relax and hold the stretch, ensuring proper breathing.
- The cable crossover machine in the weight room is a great machine to use for this stretch.

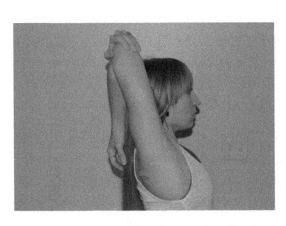

- In a standing or seated position, raise your arm over your head, bending at your elbow.
- Take your other hand and grab your elbow.
- Slowly pull your elbow back behind your head.
- Relax and hold the stretch, ensuring proper breathing.

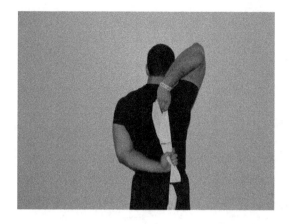

- Holding a T-Stretch strap in your hand, raise your arm over your head and bend it at your elbow. The strap should be hanging straight down behind your back.
- Grab the strap with your other hand behind your back.
- Slowly pull the band down.
- Relax and hold the stretch, ensuring proper breathing.

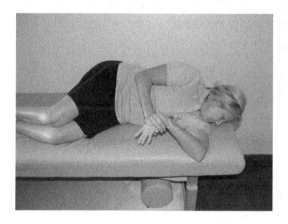

- Lying on your side, bring your arm out to a 90-degree angle. Bend your elbow and wrist also to a 90-degree angle.
- Looking straight down, place your chin on your shoulder.
- Using your other hand, grab your wrist and gently push your elbow down into the ground. Slowly push your hand down toward the floor.
- Relax and hold the stretch, ensuring proper breathing.

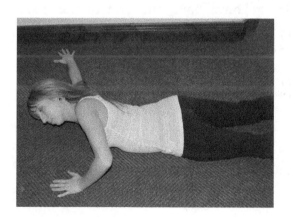

- Lying on your stomach, place your arm straight out to the side.
- Place the palm of your opposite arm under your shoulder (push up position).
- Slowly push your hand into the ground and raise your opposite shoulder off the ground.
- Relax and hold the stretch, ensuring proper breathing. **(Intermediate)**

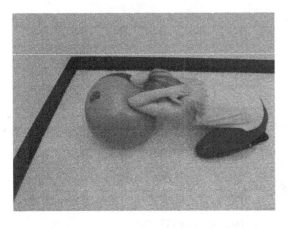

- While on your knees, place both arms straight out on a therapy ball with your thumbs up.
- Bend both arms, keeping your elbows pressed against the ball.
- Slowly push your chest down toward the ground.
- Relax and hold the stretch, ensuring proper breathing. **(Intermediate)**

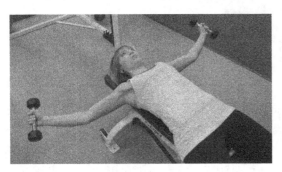

- Holding very light hand weights (3-5 pounds), lie on a bench on your back.
- Straighten your arms out to the side, palms up, and let your hands relax down toward the floor.
- Relax and hold the stretch, ensuring proper breathing. **(Intermediate)**

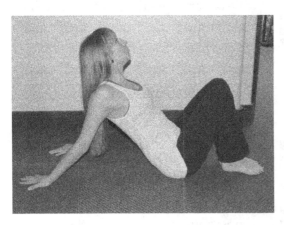

- In a seated position, bend your knees and place your arms behind you.
- Slightly raise your rear end off the ground and slowly move toward your feet until you feel a stretch.
- Lower your rear end to the floor, keeping your back straight. Don't let your chest sink down.
- Relax and hold the stretch, ensuring proper breathing. **(Intermediate)**

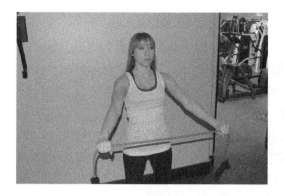 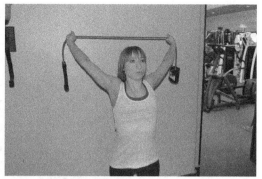

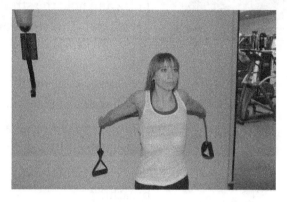

- Hold an elastic band or strap straight out in front of you.
- Slowly raise your arms up over your head and behind your back.
- Relax and hold the stretch, ensuring proper breathing.

A couple notes on this stretch:

- The width of your hand position on the band is going to depend on your flexibility.
- Always start with your hands further apart and move them in if you have to.
- The other thing you can do with this stretch is to continuously move your arms and hands back and forth over your head. **(Intermediate)**

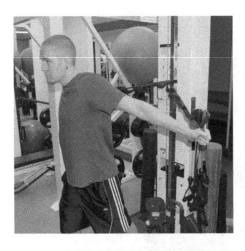

- Wrap a strap around a pole.
- In a standing position, take hold of the strap with your back to the pole. Keep your arms straight out to the side.
- Keeping your posture nice and tall, place one foot forward, and slowly move forward into the stretch. The strap should pull your hands and arms back.
- Relax and hold the stretch, ensuring proper breathing. **(Intermediate)**

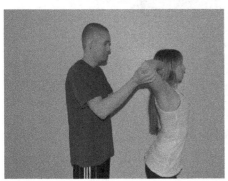

- From a standing or sitting position, interlock your hands and place them behind your head.
- Have your partner take hold of both elbows and slowly pull back.
- Relax and hold the stretch, ensuring proper breathing.
- Communicate with your partner, letting him/her know when you are feeling the stretch. **(Intermediate)**

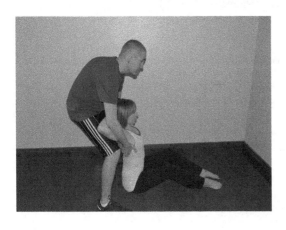

- In a seated position, interlock your hands and place them behind your head.
- Your partner will place his/her forearms over your arms and place their hands on your back.
- Have your partner slowly pull back on your arms while pushing forward on your back.
- Relax and hold the stretch, ensuring proper breathing.
- Let your partner know when you are feeling the stretch. **(Intermediate)**

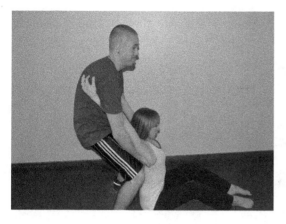

- Reach your arms above your head from a seated position on the floor.
- Have your partner place his/her arms over yours and place their hands on your back, over your shoulder blades.
- Your partner will slowly lean back while pushing your back forward.
- Relax and hold the stretch, ensuring proper breathing.
- Communicate with your partner, letting him/her know when you are feeling the stretch. **(Intermediate)**

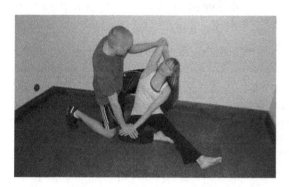

- Sitting on the ground, place your left leg straight out in front of you with your right leg bent and the bottom of your right foot against your left leg.
- Place your right hand on the back of your head with your left hand on your right knee.
- Have your partner kneel down with his/her left knee pushing slightly against your back.
- Your partner will place his/her right hand on the hand that is on your knee and his/her left hand on your elbow.
- Have your partner slowly push your elbow, causing you to lean to the side while pushing down on your knee.
- Relax and hold the stretch, ensuring proper breathing.
- Repeat on the other side.
- Communicate with your partner, letting him/her know when you feel the stretch. **(Intermediate)**

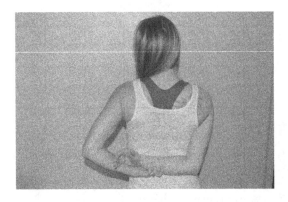

- In a standing or seated position, place your arm behind your back.
- Keeping your posture nice and tall, use your other hand and pull your arm across your back.
- Relax and hold the stretch, ensuring proper breathing. **(Intermediate)**

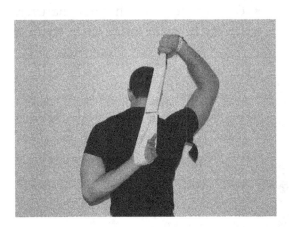

- Place your arm behind your back.
- Place your other arm over your head with your elbow bent, holding a strap in your hand.
- Grab hold of the strap behind your back and slowly pull your arm up your back.
- Relax and hold the stretch, ensuring proper breathing. **(Intermediate)**

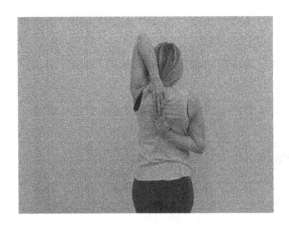

- Place one arm behind your back, and one arm bent over your head.
- Interlock your fingers and slowly pull your hands together.
- Relax and hold the stretch, ensuring proper breathing. **(Advanced)**

NECK

Tightness in the neck can be the result of sleeping in an awkward position, some sort of trauma to the neck, like a car accident, or even poor posture while sitting behind a computer at your job all day. It can create problems such as headaches and shoulder pain, as well as:

- Arthritic pain
- Dizziness
- Sinus problems
- Inability to turn your head
- Jaw pain
- Tearing of eyes

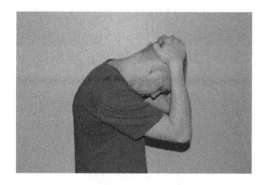

- From a standing or seated position, interlock your hands behind your head.
- Keeping your posture nice and tall, slowly pull your head down.
- Relax and hold the stretch, ensuring proper breathing.

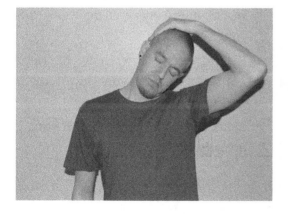

- In a standing or seated position, place your hand over the top of your head, grabbing the side of your head.
- Slowly pull your head to the side.
- Relax and hold the stretch, ensuring proper breathing.

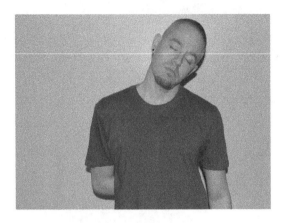

- In a standing or seated position, place your arm behind your back.
- Slowly lean your head to the other side until the stretch is felt.
- Relax and hold the stretch, ensuring proper breathing.

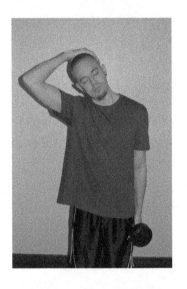

- In a standing position, hold a weight or some sort of stationary object like a table. The idea is to keep your shoulder down.
- With the other hand, slowly pull the side of your head toward the floor.
- Relax and hold the stretch, ensuring proper breathing.

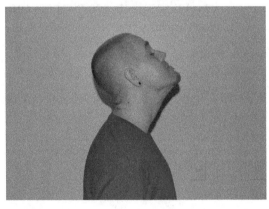

- In a standing or seated position, lean your head back.
- Extend your lower jaw forward. Think of moving your lower teeth past your upper teeth.
- Relax and hold the stretch, ensuring proper breathing.

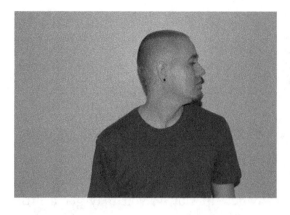

- In a standing or seated position, rotate your head to the side.
- Keep your posture nice and tall, and move your head slightly back to add a little more intensity.
- Relax and hold the stretch, ensuring proper breathing.

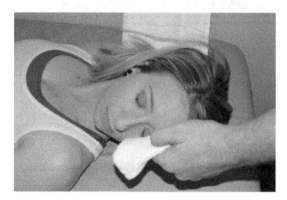

- Lying on your back, center a hand towel, folded lengthwise, under your head.
- Your partner will grab the towel on both ends and slightly raise your head off the table or floor.
- Your partner will then slowly raise one end of the towel, turning your head to the side.
- Relax and hold the stretch, then rotate to the other side. Ensure proper breathing.

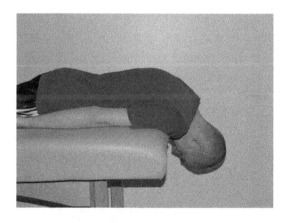

- Lie on your stomach on a massage table or bed.
- Position your shoulders at the edge, so you are far enough up so your head is allowed to hang freely.
- Relax and hold the stretch, ensuring proper breathing.
- Due to blood rushing to your head, get up slowly, you may get a little dizzy. **(Intermediate)**

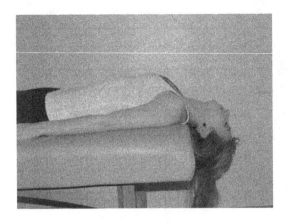

- Lie on your back on a massage table or bed.
- Position your shoulders at the edge, so you are far enough up so your head is allowed to hang back freely.
- Relax and hold the stretch, ensuring proper breathing.
- Due to blood rushing to your head, get up slowly, you may get a little dizzy. **(Intermediate)**

DYNAMIC STRETCHES

Ex-MLB All-Star Erik Hanson mentioned something to me that I like to share with all my clients. He told me that when he was pitching, he warmed up to throw; he didn't throw to warm up. The same thing goes with his amateur golfing career—he warms up to hit balls; he doesn't hit balls to warm up. I witness Erik performing many dynamic stretches every day he plays golf. I placed these stretches in a category all by themselves primarily because they typically involve stretching and using more than one muscle group. They involve active movements that are not only sport specific, but everyday life specific movements that we do every day...or should. I encourage you to add these to your daily routine, but move slowly and hold on to something for stability if needed. Dynamic stretches are a perfect addition to any warm-up or exercise program, but, as with anything, there are several things to keep in mind:

- Perform a 5-10 minute aerobic workout prior to your dynamic stretches.
- Use a foam roller to help release adhesions in the muscles.
- Perform each exercise 10-15 times.
- Ensure proper body posture.
- Perform the dynamic stretches that most closely resemble your daily activities.
- Slowly increase your speed and range of motion as you progress.
- Focus on your breathing.

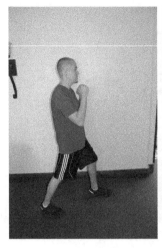 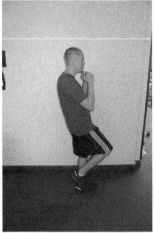 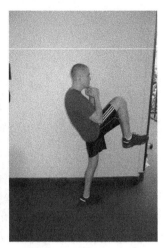

- Keeping your hands up, stand with one foot back with toes pointed forward.
- Your weight should transfer totally to your front foot as you begin to move your back knee forward.
- Staying under control, raise your back knee as high as you can.
- You should feel a slight stretch (in the hip and possibly even in the hamstrings closer to your glutes if you are tighter) within the leg lifted off the ground.
- Ensure proper breathing and repeat 10-15 times.
- Hold on to something stable for balance and support if needed.

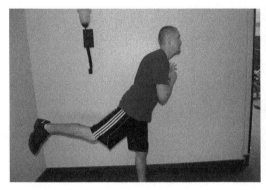 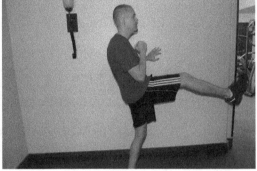

- Standing next to something stable for support and balance, swing your leg forward to get a stretch in your hamstring.
- Immediately swing your leg back behind you, stretching your hip flexors.
- Ensure proper breathing and repeat this stretch 10-15 times with each leg.
- Hold on to something stable for support and balance if needed.

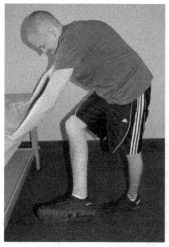 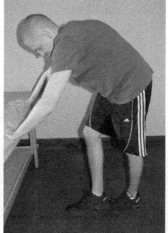 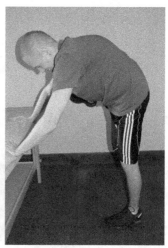

- Hold on to a stable object for support and balance.
- Standing approximately 2-3 feet away from support, bring one leg forward.
- Swing your leg across your body and out to the side, safely trying to get as much movement in your hip as possible. You will feel this on the inside of your leg as well as in your glutes.
- Ensure proper breathing and repeat this stretch 10-15 times.

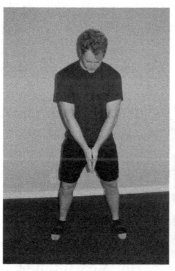 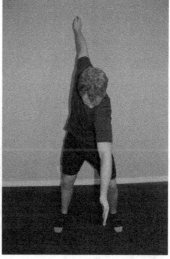

- Stand with your feet shoulder-width apart with the palms of your hands together out in front of you (like a golf stance).
- Keeping your arms straight, slowly turn to the right side, bringing your right arm behind and above your head. Keep your left arm in the starting position.

- Return to the starting position and repeat to the left side.
- I like to do this stretch in a constant motion, performing 10-15 repetitions. I then hold the position of the last stretch on each side.

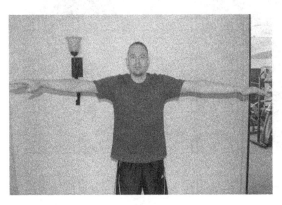

- Keeping your posture tall in a standing or seated position, lift your arms straight out to the sides.
- Begin doing forward circles with your arms. Perform 15-20 circles, and then do backward circles 15-20 repetitions.
- I also like to change the size of the circles from time to time.

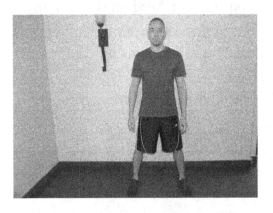

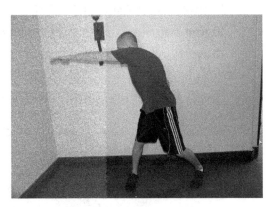

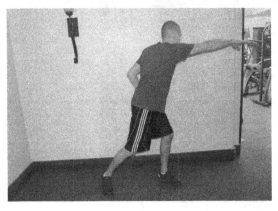

- Stand with your feet approximately shoulder-width apart.
- Turn your body and, with your left hand, reach as far as you can to your right side, then immediately turn back and reach with your right hand as far as you can to your left side.
- This stretch can be felt all the way down the side of your reaching arm and down into the lower back.
- Ensure proper breathing and repeat 10-15 times on each side.

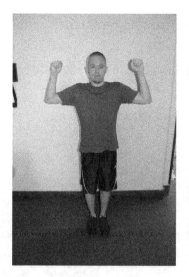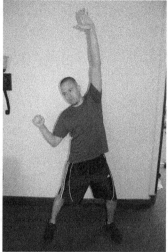

- Start with your feet together and both hands up with your elbows at shoulder height.
- Step out past shoulder-width with your left foot and raise your left arm high above your head. Return to the starting position and repeat on your right side, each time ensuring you are reaching as high into the sky as you possibly can. Don't get lazy.
- You should feel this stretch all the way down the side of your outstretched arm.
- Ensure proper breathing and repeat 10-15 times on each side.

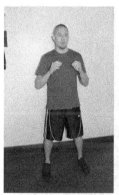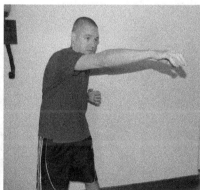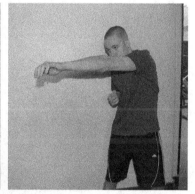

- Keeping your hands up, start with your feet approximately shoulder-width apart.
- Rotate your body and push your hand straight out in front, really trying to reach as far as you can in front of your body. I always tell my clients to visualize something they need to grab and then pull it back in. Repeat on the other side.

- This stretch should be felt in the side of the outreached arm and down into the lower back.
- Ensure proper breathing and repeat 10-15 times on each side.

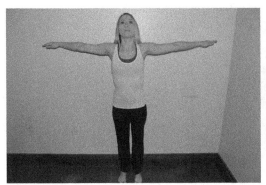 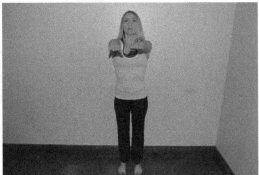

- In a standing or seated position, place your arms at shoulder height.
- Keeping your posture nice and tall, bring your hands in together and then right back out.
- Move slowly as you begin, adding just a little more speed as you warm up. When doing this stretch, I focus on separating my shoulder blades when my hands are in front and squeezing my shoulder blades together as I bring my hands back.
- Ensure proper breathing and repeat 10-15 times.

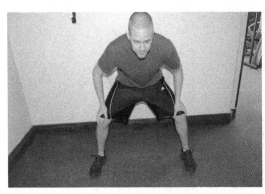 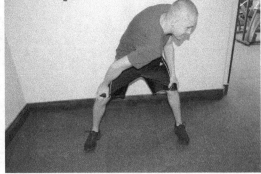

- Start with your feet a little wider than shoulder-width apart.
- Slightly squat down and place your hands on your knees.
- Slowly turn your right shoulder in toward your left knee as you slightly push your right knee out.

- Repeat to the other side.
- You should feel this stretch in between your shoulder blades and down the center of your back. People who are tight may also feel this in the groin.
- Ensure proper breathing and repeat 10-15 times on each side.

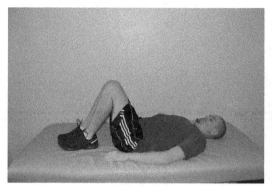 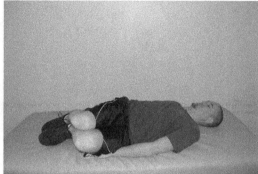

- Lying on your back, bend your knees and place your feet flat on the floor/bed.
- Slowly move your knees to the side, keeping them together until you feel the stretch.
- Return to the starting position and repeat on the other side.
- Ensure proper breathing and repeat 15-20 times each direction.
- This stretch is great for individuals with arthritic hips. It can also be a great move for people with lower back issues.

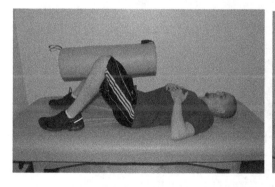 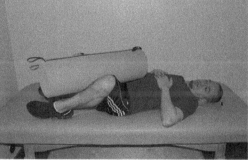

- Lying on your back, bend your knees and place your feet flat on the floor/bed.
- Place something between your knees like a pillow or ball. Squeezing the object, slowly move your knees to the side until you feel the stretch.

- Return to the starting position and repeat on the other side.
- Ensure proper breathing and repeat 15-20 times in each direction.

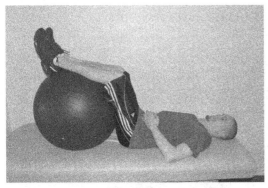 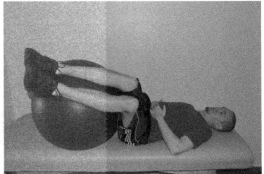

- Lying on your back, place your legs on top of a therapy ball.
- Slowly rotate the ball to the side until you feel the stretch.
- Move back to the starting position and repeat the stretch to the other side.
- Ensure proper breathing and repeat the stretch 15-20 times in each direction.

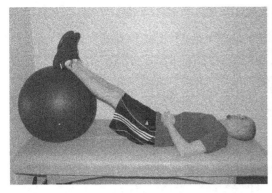 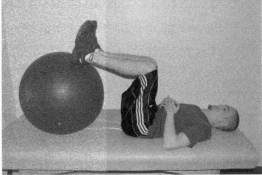

- Lying on your back, place your heels near the center of a therapy ball.
- Bending your knees, slowly pull the ball in toward your rear end until you feel the stretch.
- Move the ball back to the starting position and repeat.
- Ensure proper breathing and repeat the stretch 15-20 times.

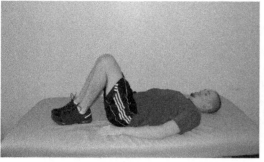 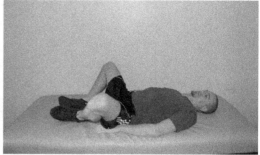

- Lying on your back, bend your knees and place your feet flat on the floor/bed.
- Slowly spread your knees apart from each other until the stretch is felt.
- Return to the starting position and repeat the stretch.
- Ensure proper breathing and repeat the stretch 10-15 times.
- This dynamic stretch is great for the muscles in the inner leg. It is also another great move to do for arthritic hips as well as lower back pain.

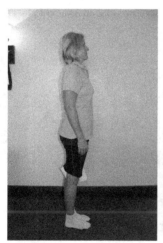 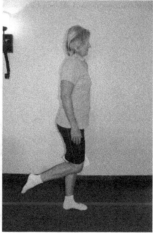

- In a standing position, place a folded hand towel between your knees and hold it there.
- Hold on to a stationary object for balance!
- Slowly raise your foot up behind you, keeping the towel between your knees. Return your foot back to the floor.
- Repeat 10-15 times.
- Relax and ensure proper breathing throughout the entire movement.

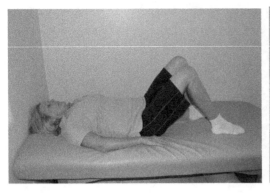 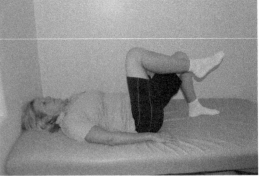

- Lying on your back, bend both knees.
- Slowly raise your knee up, keeping the same angle in your leg.
- Repeat 10-15 times.
- Relax and maintain proper breathing throughout the entire movement.

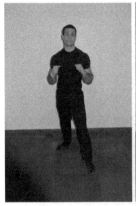 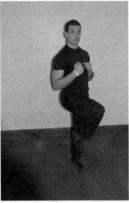 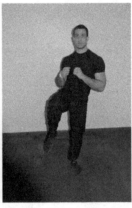 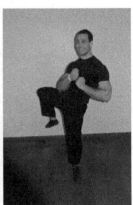

- Stand with one foot behind you, keeping your hands up.
- Bring your back leg up and to the opposite side.
- Fan your knee up and across your body, then back to the starting position.
- Ensure proper breathing and repeat 10-15 times with each leg. **(Intermediate)**

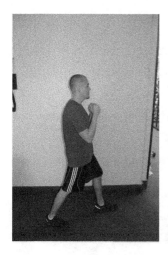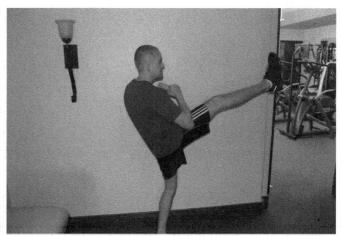

- With both hands up, stand with one foot back with toes pointed forward.
- Your weight will begin to move to your forward foot as your back leg kicks forward and up.
- This stretch allows you to stand in place as you focus on bringing your foot back to the starting position, or you can do this moving forward. As you do your front kick, bring the leg straight down in front of you and repeat the front kick with your other leg.
- You will feel this stretch in the hamstrings of your kicking leg.
- Ensure proper breathing and repeat this stretch 10-15 times with each leg.
- Hold on to something stable for support and balance if needed. **(Intermediate)**

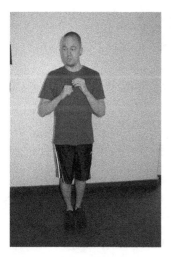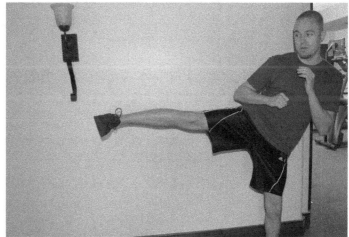

- With both hands up, stand with both feet together.
- When raising your right leg, start by placing your weight on your left foot. Staying under control, raise your leg up to the side as high as you can get it. Slowly lower your leg back to the starting position.
- You will feel this stretch again in your hip as well as the inside of your leg and your groin muscles.
- Ensure proper breathing and repeat this stretch 10-15 times. **(Intermediate)**

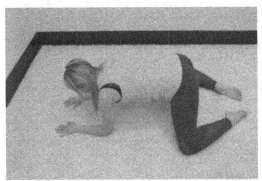 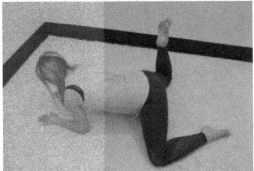

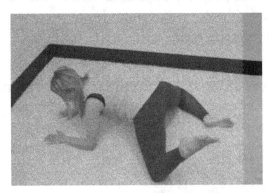

- Get down on your hands and knees, spreading your knees as far apart as you can with your feet remaining on the floor. You should feel a little stretch on the inside of your legs.
- Lean forward and rotate your right leg on your knee, bringing your foot off the floor, stretching your hip.
- As you return your right leg back to the starting position, rotate your left leg up.
- Repeat this stretch 10-15 times in each direction. **(Intermediate)**

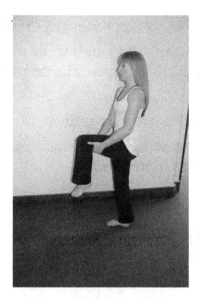 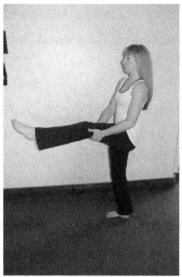

- Begin by standing with your feet together. Raise one leg and grasp with both hands under your leg, just above the knee. Try to keep your knee approximately at belt level.

- Ensuring proper balance, straighten your leg.

- You will feel this stretch on the back of your leg in your hamstrings. You will also begin to feel the muscles in your thigh working as well.

- Ensure proper breathing and repeat the stretch 10-15 times. **(Intermediate)**

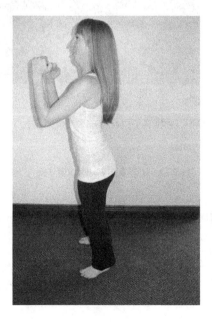 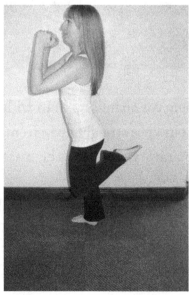

- Keeping your hands up, stand with your feet approximately 6 inches apart.
- Raise your leg off the ground and attempt to hit your rear end with your heel. Slowly lower your leg to the starting position. Repeat with your opposite leg.
- You will feel this stretch in your thighs (quadriceps).
- Ensure proper breathing and repeat this stretch 10-15 times.
- If you are more advanced, speed up the process by jogging in place while trying to touch your heels to your rear end. **(Intermediate)**

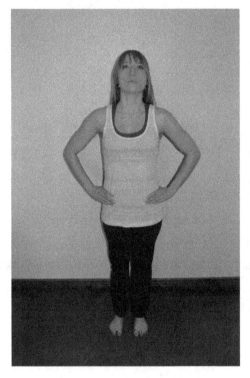
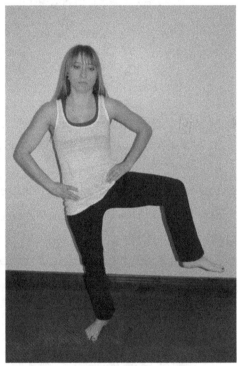

- Keeping your hands up, start with your feet together.
- Lift your knee straight up in front of you.
- As you raise your knee as high as it can comfortably go, swing your knee out to the side.
- Slowly lower your leg back down to the starting position and repeat on the other side.
- This is a great one to develop better hip movement
- Ensure proper breathing and repeat this stretch 10-15 times. **(Intermediate)**

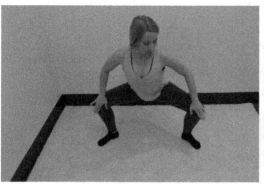 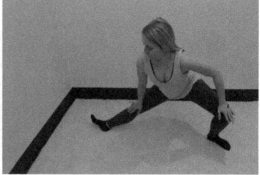

- Start with your feet approximately twice your shoulder width
- Squat down and place your hands on the inside of your knees.
- Keeping your back straight and head up, lunge down toward the left side. Keep your knee over your heel and point the toes of your straightened leg up.
- Return back to the starting position and repeat on the other side.
- This stretch should be felt in the muscles on the inside of your straight leg.
- Ensure proper breathing and repeat 10-15 times on each side. **(Intermediate)**

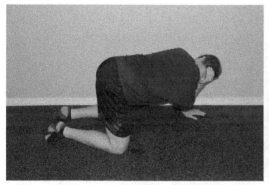 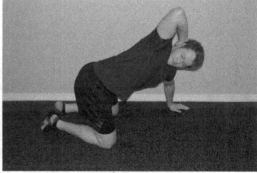

- Starting on your hands and knees, place one hand behind your head.
- Slowly turn your body so that your elbow moves in toward your other arm.
- Rotate in toward your other arm as far as you can comfortably go, feeling the stretch behind your shoulder blade down to your lower back.
- Rotate out, trying to point your elbow up at the ceiling, working on getting that full range of motion in your back.
- Ensure proper breathing and repeat 15-20 times on each side. **(Intermediate)**

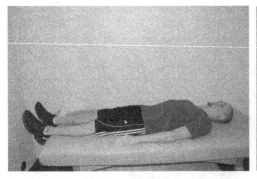 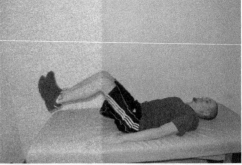

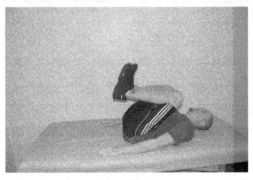

- Lie on your back with your knees and feet together. Keep your arms to your side.
- Raise your knees all the way to your chest.
- Slowly return back to the starting position.
- Ensure proper breathing and repeat 15-20 times.
- This move can put a tremendous amount of pressure on your lower back. Use caution if you have back problems. **(Intermediate)**

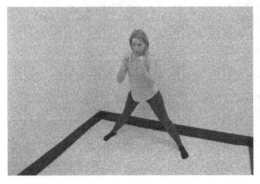 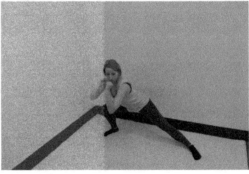

- Keeping your arms out in front of you, stand with your feet approximately twice your shoulder width.

- Keeping your posture nice and tall, look straight ahead. Squat down toward your right leg, thinking about keeping your posterior back. Keep your knee above your heel; don't let it get past your toes.
- Stand back up to the full starting position and repeat on the left side.
- This should be felt on the inside of the straight leg and can also be felt in the hamstring and glutes of the bent leg.
- Ensure proper breathing and repeat 10-15 times on each side.
- If your knees move past your toes, you can put tremendous pressure on the knees. **(Intermediate)**

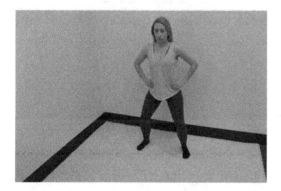
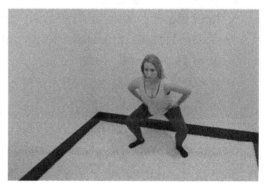

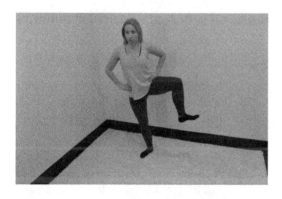

- Begin with your feet a little wider than shoulder-width apart.
- Squat down until you feel the stretch.
- Return to your standing position and bring your knee up. Work on bringing it up higher and higher as you do more reps.
- Lower your leg and repeat the process, this time picking up your other leg.
- Ensure proper breathing and repeat 10-15 times on each side. **(Intermediate)**

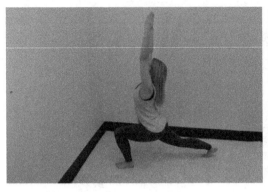 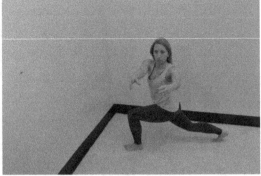

- Keeping your arms straight above you, stand with your feet together.
- Keeping your posture tall with your head up, take a large step forward and squat straight down. Keeping your back leg straight, ensure your front knee doesn't pass your toes.
- Lowering your arms in front of you, rotate your upper body toward the side of your forward foot.
- Keeping your balance, slowly return to the starting position and repeat with the other leg.
- You should feel this stretch in the thigh and hip flexors of the back leg and into the lower back.
- Ensure proper breathing and repeat 10-15 times on each side. **(Intermediate)**

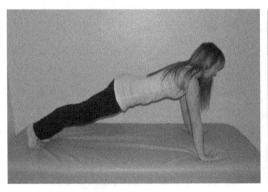 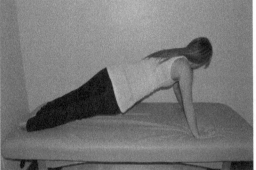

- Begin in a push-up position.
- Slowly rotate your hips to the side until you feel a stretch in your torso.
- Return back to the starting position and repeat in the other direction.
- Ensure proper breathing and repeat 10-15 times on each side. **(Intermediate)**

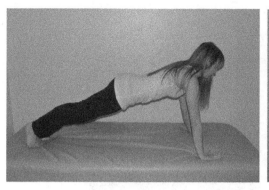 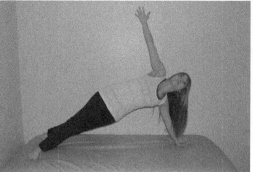

- Begin in a push-up position.
- Rotate your left hip to the side, bringing your right hand off the floor. Slowly work your way to raising your right hand straight up toward the ceiling.
- Return to the starting position and repeat on the other side.
- Ensure proper breathing and repeat 10-15 times. **(Intermediate)**

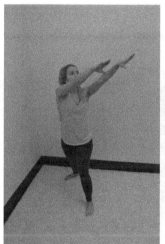 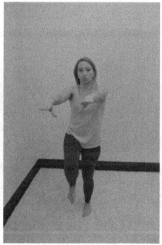 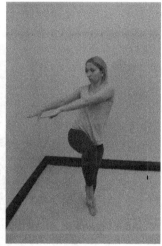

- Begin with your left leg forward and your right leg back with your arms reaching out toward your left side.
- Bring your right knee forward as you rotate your upper body toward the right side.
- With your right knee now approximately waist height, rotate your upper body all the way to the right side with your hands even with your hips.
- Return to the starting position and repeat 10-15 times. Switch to the other side.
- Ensure proper breathing. **(Intermediate)**

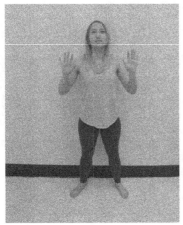 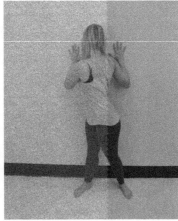

- Stand with your back approximately one foot away from a wall.
- With your feet shoulder-width apart and your palms up, slowly turn your body and try to place your hands on the wall. DON'T FORCE IT!
- Repeat the stretch to the other side.
- With this stretch, you can hold the position, or you can slowly turn from side to side and just touch the wall performing 10-15 repetitions. **(Advanced)**

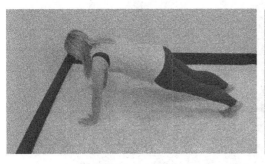 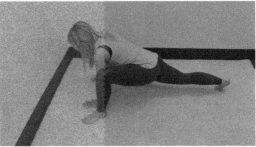

- Begin in a push-up position.
- Slowly raise your leg and place your foot up by your hand.
- Keep your hips raised, don't let them sink toward the ground.
- Slowly return to the starting position and repeat with the other side.
- You should feel this in the hip flexor of the straight leg and in the glutes and hamstrings of the bent leg.
- Ensure proper breathing and repeat 10-15 times on each side.
- If you feel a pinching sensation in the hip flexors of the bent knee, this can be a great indicator that those muscles are tight. **(Advanced)**

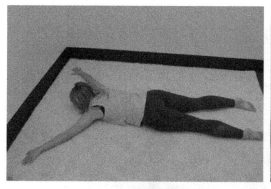
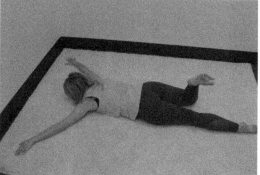
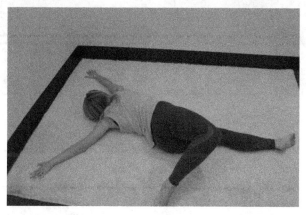

- Lie on your stomach on the floor with your legs and arms spread apart.
- Bend a knee and slowly try to touch your feet to the ground on the opposite side of your body.
- Slowly return to the starting position and repeat on the other side.
- This stretch is a favorite of mine because you may feel a stretch in many different areas. You can feel this in the lower back, in your hip flexors, as well as in your latissimus dorsi.
- Ensure proper breathing and repeat 10-15 times on each side.
- This one is not always recommended for people with lower back issues. Take care and move slowly on this stretch. **(Advanced)**

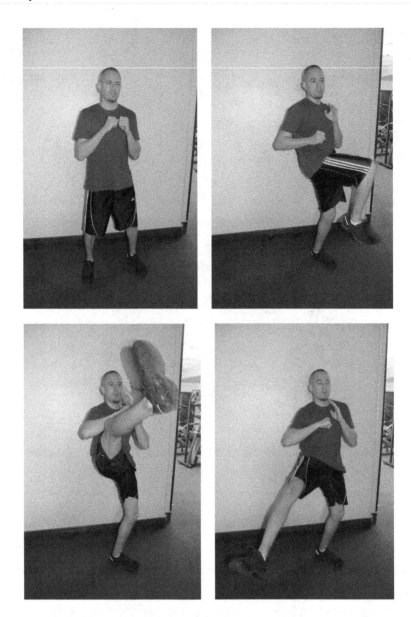

- Begin by standing with your feet shoulder-width apart with your hands up.
- Shifting your weight to your left foot, lift your right leg, bending your knee, and bring it across your body to the left side.
- Straighten your leg, kicking your right foot out and up and then back across to the right side of your body. This movement should be in the shape of a rainbow, starting low, reaching your highest point straight in front of you, and returning low at your starting point. **(Advanced)**

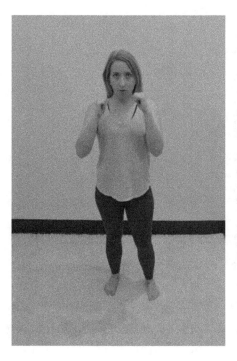
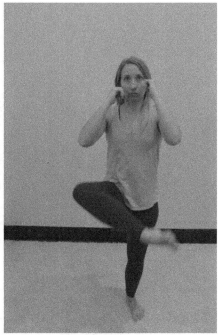

- Keeping your hands up, start with your feet approximately 6 inches apart.
- Begin this movement by lifting your knee up. As you lift your knee, begin to bring your foot in toward your other leg and think of pushing your foot up toward your belt line.
- This movement can be done slowly; however, to be more effective, you can do this like you are running in place.
- This movement is great for the muscles in the hip.
- Ensure proper breathing and repeat this stretch 10-15 times. **(Advanced)**

BALL STRETCHING ROUTINE

I absolutely love using the ball in my stretching routine. Not only can the ball break up the monotony of your normal stretching routine, it can provide you ways to stretch and strengthen muscles that you probably never thought about. I would suggest this program to individuals with more than average balance and flexibility, however, you can use the wall or other stationary object to maintain balance. Within the program you will hit muscles in your hamstrings, hip flexors, glutes, abdominals, upper back, chest, and your lats.

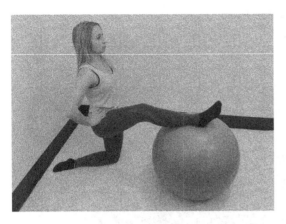

HAMSTRING

- Place your heel on the center of the ball and lower yourself so your other knee is on the ground (use a wall or other stationary object for support if necessary).
- Keep your leg slightly bent and your posture nice and tall. Slowly move the ball towards you.

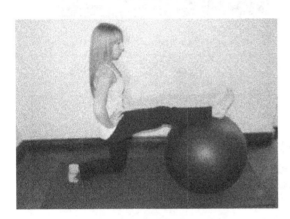

- Place your heel on the center of the ball and lower yourself so your other knee is on the ground (use a wall or other stationary object for support if necessary).
- Focus on keeping your leg straight while keeping your posture nice and tall.

HIP FLEXOR

- Straddling the ball, place your shin and knee on top of the ball.
- Keeping your posture nice and tall, bend your front knee and lower your body toward the ground.
- Push your knee and shin into the ball as you lower your hip flexor down.

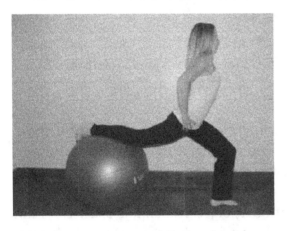

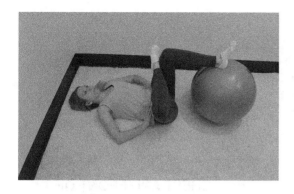

GLUTES

- Lying on your back, place your leg straight out on top of the ball.
- Place your ankle just above your knee.
- Slowly bend your knee and pull the ball in toward your body until you feel a stretch.

LOWER BACK

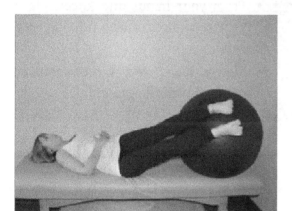

- Lying on your back, place your feet on top of a therapy ball.
- Use your feet to turn the ball to the side, rotating your legs to the side as well.
- For traction, do this with shoes on or with bare feet. To get a better stretch, try placing your feet further to the side of the ball from the starting position.

ABDOMINALS

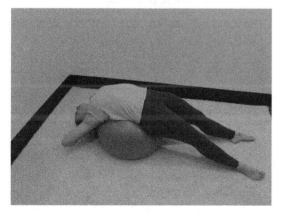

- Begin by sitting on a therapy ball. Slowly roll yourself down into a lying position.
- Position yourself so that your mid back is centered on the ball.
- Keeping your legs straight, extend your arms over your head or place them behind your head and slowly relax your body to take the shape of the ball.

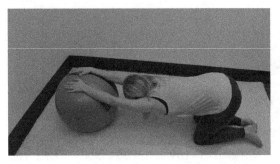

UPPER BACK

- While on your knees, place your arms straight out with your palms down on a therapy ball.
- Keeping your arms straight, slowly lower your chest to the ground.

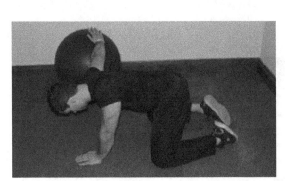

CHEST AND FRONT OF SHOULDER

- From your hands and knees, place your straightened arm on a therapy ball.
- Slowly lower the same shoulder down toward the ground.

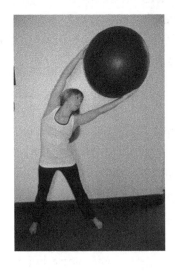

LOWER BACK AND SIDE OF UPPER BODY

- Stand with your feet approximately shoulder-width apart.
- Holding on to a therapy ball, extend your arms over your head.
- Keeping your posture nice and tall, lean to the side and focus on pushing the ball up and away from your body.

Stretching Programs

I am asked all the time what my favorite stretches are, what I would recommend for certain ailments, and what someone should do for a specific sport or activity. The following pages contain specific stretches that I believe can help you in these situations. Please remember that these are just suggestions and are based on my experiences with people in these areas. They obviously don't take into account your self-evaluation; however, they are well-rounded programs that can benefit most people.

I would urge you to try new programs, but make sure you consider your evaluation and stretching level. If you are a beginner, don't do an advanced stretch, much less an advanced routine! Stretching can cause a level of discomfort, but don't continue a stretch that is actually causing you pain. I have said it before, but make sure that you have correct posture and that you are breathing correctly during each stretch. Occasionally you will notice yourself tensing up, which is usually caused by holding your breath or even doing a stretch you are not entirely comfortable doing. Try to focus on totally letting your body go during each stretch. As you are breathing in, focus on that air you are breathing rushing to the muscle you are stretching.

Each program has a series of pictures of stretches with instructions for each stretch that I would recommend. I challenge you to stretch every day in the morning, after your workout, or before you go to bed. I assure you that if you make this a part of your daily routine so that it becomes a habit, your body will thank you for it!

DYNAMIC STRETCHING FOR SPORTS

As I was going through all my programs for sports, I noticed that they were just too long. I want to make sure you are totally focused on your routine and when it becomes too overwhelming, your focus my wander. In order to keep you fully focused on what you need to be working on, I decided to put together a general sport specific dynamic stretching program that can be used by anyone who is wanting to perform better, regardless of what sport you are playing. Remember what you are doing this for, make sure you are focusing on your posture and constantly pushing yourself to get better. Later in this section I will present the more relaxing passive and static routines for each specific sport.

HAMSTRING

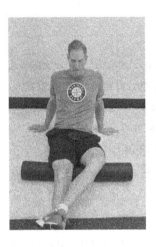

- Start by sitting on the floor with your knees slightly bent.
- Slide the foam roller underneath your legs and place it against your hamstrings (the large muscle group above the knee).
- Place your hands behind you and lift your rear off the floor.
- Slowly roll lengthwise up and down the muscle.
- Remember, when you find those tight areas, hold for 15-30 seconds.

GLUTES

- Sit on the foam roller with your hands on the ground behind you.
- Bend both knees, keeping knees and feet together.
- Rotate your knees to the side, stabilizing yourself with the one arm that you are leaning toward. Slowly roll the muscles in your hips.
- The second picture shows the advanced version. Start by placing your right ankle on your straightened left leg, just above the knee. Ensure you are leaning on your right arm.

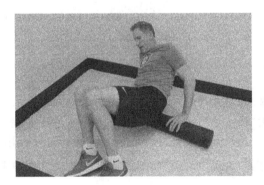
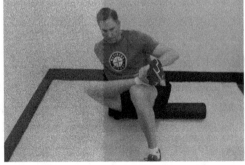

- Keep your ankle stabilized and bend your left knee.
- Slowly roll up and down your hip. Take note that you are now rolling a muscle that is actually getting stretched at the same time. This will be a very tender area when you first begin.

HIP FLEXOR

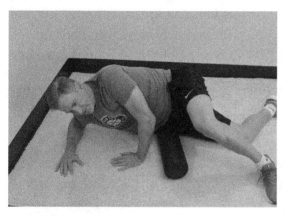

- Place the roller on the group of muscles just under your hip bone.
- If you are working on your left side, your left leg will be straight. Bend your right leg at a 90- degree angle and place your right foot on the ground.
- Lean slightly to the left side and do short movements up and down your hip flexor muscles.

UPPER BACK

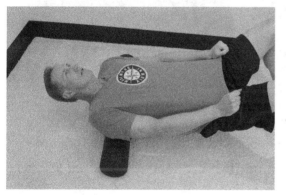

- Sit on the floor with the roller behind you and perpendicular to your body.
- Keeping your knees bent, lay back, placing the roller just above the midline.
- Raise your pelvis off the floor and slowly roll up and down your spine, ensuring that you do not take the roller lower than the rib cage.
- Relax your body and take the shape of the roller.

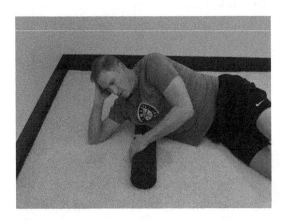

LATISIMUS DORSI

- Laying your side on the floor, place the roller underneath you just below your armpit.
- Support your head with your hand.
- Rest the leg of the side you are lying on while using your upper leg and arm to slowly move your body up and down the big muscle on the outside of your upper back.

HAMSTRING

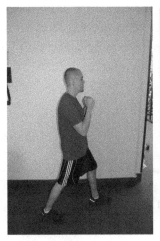
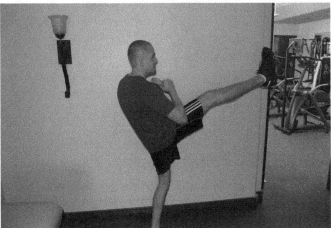

- With both hands up, stand with one foot back with toes pointed forward.
- Your weight will begin to move to your forward foot as your back leg kicks forward and up.
- This stretch allows you to stand in place as you focus on bringing your foot back to the starting position, or you can do this moving forward. As you do your front kick, bring the leg straight down in front of you and repeat the front kick with your other leg.
- Hold on to something stable for support and balance if needed. Repeat 10-15 times.

GLUTES AND ADDUCTORS

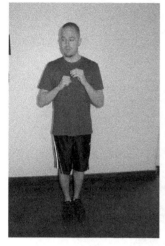 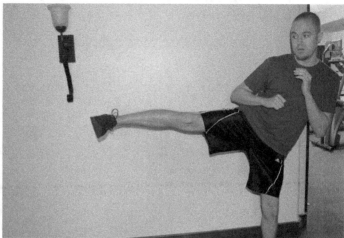

- With both hands up, stand with both feet together.
- When raising your right leg, start by placing your weight on your left foot. Staying under control, raise your leg up to the side as high as you can get it. Slowly lower your leg back to the starting position. Repeat 10-15 times each direction.

ADDUCTORS AND HIPS

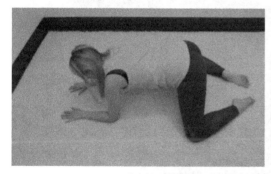 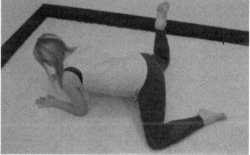

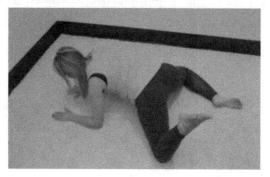

- Get down on your hands and knees, spreading your knees as far apart as you can with your feet remaining on the floor. You should feel a little stretch on the inside of your legs.
- Lean forward and rotate your right leg on your knee, bringing your foot off the floor, stretching your hip.
- As you return your right leg back to the starting position, rotate your left leg up.
- Repeat this stretch 10-15 times in each direction.

THIGHS

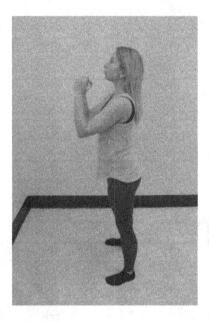 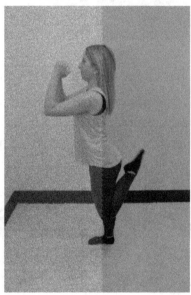

- Keeping your hands up, stand with your feet approximately 6 inches apart.
- Raise your leg off the ground and attempt to hit your rear end with your heel. Slowly lower your leg to the starting position. Repeat with your opposite leg.
- Ensure proper breathing and repeat this stretch 10-15 times.
- If you are more advanced, speed up the process by jogging in place while trying to touch your heels to your rear end.

INNER THIGH

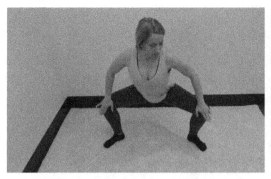 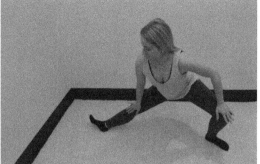

- Start with your feet approximately twice your shoulder width
- Squat down and place your hands on the inside of your knees.
- Keeping your back straight and head up, lunge down toward the left side. Keep your knee over your heel and point the toes of your straightened leg up.
- Return back to the starting position and repeat on the other side.
- This stretch should be felt in the muscles on the inside of your straight leg. Repeat 10-15 times.

UPPER AND LOWER BACK

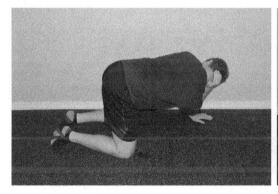 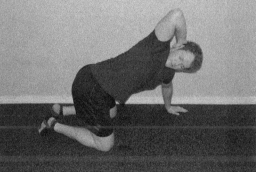

- Starting on your hands and knees, place one hand behind your head.
- Slowly turn your body so that your elbow moves in toward your other arm.
- Rotate in toward your other arm as far as you can comfortably go, feeling the stretch behind your shoulder blade down to your lower back.
- Rotate out, trying to point your elbow up at the ceiling, working on getting that full range of motion in your back. Repeat 10-15 times each direction.

THIGH, HIP FLEXOR, AND LOWER BACK

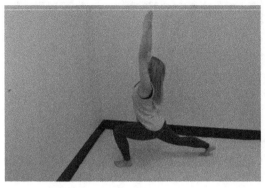 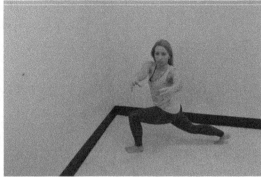

- Keeping your arms straight above you, stand with your feet together.
- Keeping your posture tall with your head up, take a large step forward and squat straight down. Keeping your back leg straight, ensure your front knee doesn't pass your toes.
- Lowering your arms in front of you, rotate your upper body toward the side of your forward foot.
- Keeping your balance, slowly return to the starting position and repeat with the other leg.

HIP FLEXOR, GLUTES, AND HAMSTRING

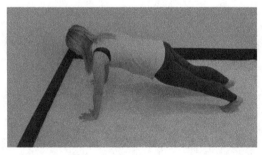 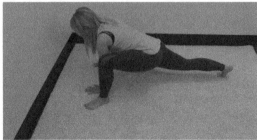

- Begin in a push up position.
- Slowly raise your leg and place your foot up by your hand.
- Keep your hips raised, don't let them sink toward the ground.
- Slowly return to the starting position and repeat with the other side. Repeat 10-15 times.
- If you feel a pinching sensation in the hip flexors of the bent knee, this can be a great indicator that those muscles are tight.

LOWER BACK, HIP FLEXORS, AND UPPER BACK

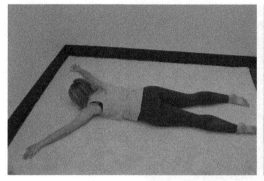 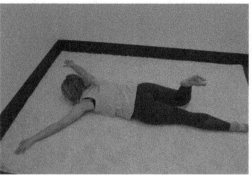

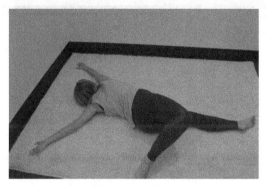

- Lie on your stomach on the floor with your legs and arms spread apart.
- Bend a knee and slowly try to touch your feet to the ground on the opposite side of your body.
- Slowly return to the starting position and repeat on the other side.
- This stretch is a favorite of mine because you may feel a stretch in many different areas. You can feel this in the lower back, in your hip flexors, as well as in your latisimus dorsi.
- This one is not always recommended for people with lower back issues. Take care and move slowly on this stretch. Repeat 10-15 times.

CHEST AND SHOULDERS

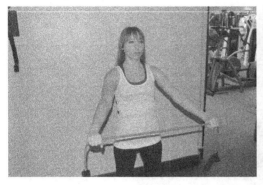 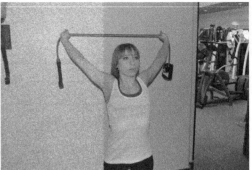

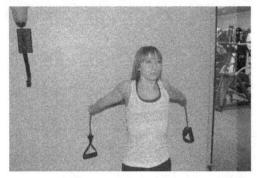

- Hold an elastic band or strap straight out in front of you.
- Slowly raise your arms up over your head and behind your back.
- Relax and hold the stretch, ensuring proper breathing.
- A couple notes on this stretch: the width of your hand position on the band is going to depend on your flexibility. Always start with your hands further apart and move them in if you have to. The other thing you can do with this stretch is to continuously move your arms and hands back and forth over your head.

My Favorite Stretches

I am asked all the time what my favorite stretches are. So, I have put together three different programs containing my favorite stretches. With the following three programs, I provide you a well-rounded program that targets some of the tighter areas I find when I am working with my clients. This first program is wonderful for people looking to work on their lower body and back.

MY FAVORITE STRETCHES (PROGRAM #1)

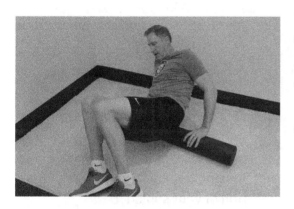

GLUTES

- Sit on the foam roller with your hands on the ground behind you.
- Bend both knees, keeping knees and feet together.
- Rotate your knees to the side, stabilizing yourself with the one arm and slowly roll the muscles in your hips.

IT BAND

- Start by laying the outside of your leg on the roller.
- Place your leg on top of the leg you are rolling.
- Once you feel comfortable, slowly roll lengthwise up and down. Find those tender areas and hold for 15-30 seconds.

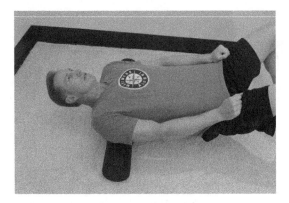

UPPER BACK

- Sit on the floor with the roller behind you and perpendicular to your body.
- Keeping your knees bent, lay back, placing the roller just above the midline.
- Raise your pelvis off the floor and slowly roll up and down your spine, ensuring that you do not take the roller lower than the rib cage.
- Relax your body and take the shape of the roller.

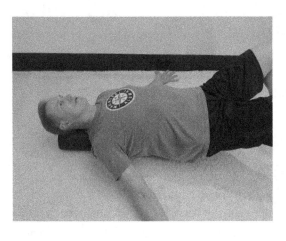

BACK AND CHEST

- Lie on the roller lengthwise with your head, upper back, and tailbone supported. Bend both knees and keep your feet flat on the floor for support.
- Draw your navel in and perform a pelvic tilt, laying your lower back on the roller.
- Now, bring your hands straight out into a T-shape position. In this position, you will feel a stretch in the upper back, chest, and the front portion of your shoulders.

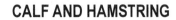

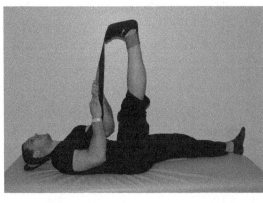

CALF AND HAMSTRING

- Lying flat on your back, place the TStretch strap around your ankle and up the bottom of your foot.
- Bring your leg straight up and pull back and down on the strap.
- Relax and hold the stretch, ensuring proper breathing.

HAMSTRING

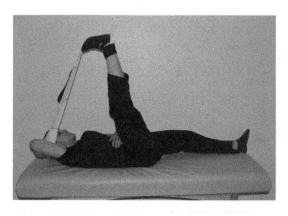

- Lying on your back, place the TStretch strap around your ankle and up the bottom of your foot.
- Keeping your leg straight, pull your leg towards you.
- Relax and hold the stretch, ensuring proper breathing.

HIP FLEXOR

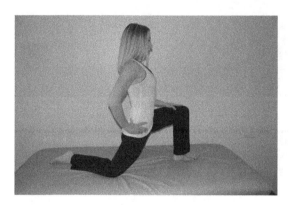

- Get down on both knees and place one foot forward in a lunge position.
- Take your weight down and forward, keeping your posture nice and tall.
- Relax and hold the stretch, ensuring proper breathing.

THIGH, HIP FLEXOR, AND HAMSTRING

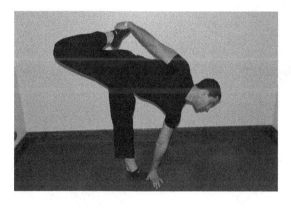

- In a standing position, grab a foot and pull it up to your rear end.
- Keeping hold of your foot, slowly lean forward and touch your hand to the floor.
- Keep your posture nice and tall.
- Relax and hold the position, ensuring proper breathing.

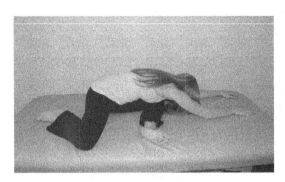

GLUTES

- In a seated position, bend one leg and place it behind you and bend your forward leg to a 90-degree angle.
- Keeping your posture nice and tall, lean forward toward your knee.
- Relax and hold the stretch, ensuring proper breathing.

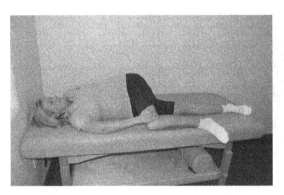

GLUTES AND LOWER BACK

- Lie on your side, bend your top leg and place it at a 90-degree angle.
- Slowly push your top shoulder back to the ground, holding your upper knee down to the floor.
- Relax and hold the stretch, ensuring proper breathing.

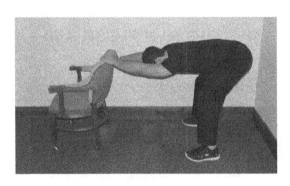

UPPER BACK

- In a standing position, place your hands on the back of a chair.
- Slowly move your chest down toward the ground keeping your hips up.
- Relax and hold the stretch, ensuring proper breathing.

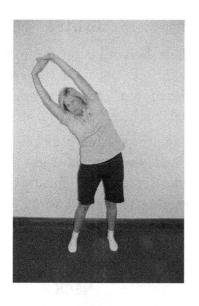

SIDE OF ABDOMINALS AND LOWER BACK

- Stand with your feet approximately shoulder-width apart.
- Interlock your fingers and raise your arms over your head.
- Keeping your posture nice and tall, lean to the side and focus on pushing the palms of your hands up and out away from your body.
- Relax and hold the stretch, ensuring proper breathing.

MY FAVORITE STRETCHES (PROGRAM #2)

This program is a little more advanced and focuses a little more on balance as well. This is a great program for an individual who is looking for more mobility in the hips and lower back. I have also added a great stretch for your chest and your upper back for rotation. I love this routine for anyone looking to add more rotation to their spine and golf swing.

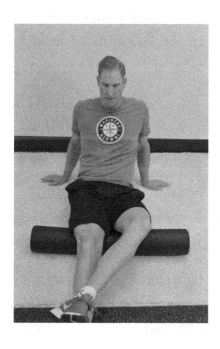

HAMSTRING

- Start by sitting on the floor with your knees slightly bent.
- Slide the foam roller underneath your legs and place it against your hamstrings (the large muscle group above the knee).
- Place your hands behind you and lift your rear off the floor.
- Slowly roll lengthwise up and down the muscle.
- Remember, when you find those tight areas, hold for 15- 30 seconds.

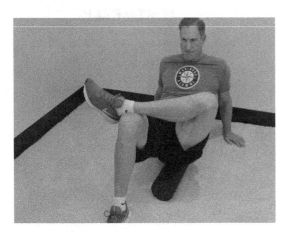

GLUTES

- Start by sitting on the roller with both knees bent. If you are rolling the left hip, lean to that side and stabilize yourself with your left arm.

- Begin by placing your left ankle on your straightened right leg, just above the knee. Ensure you are leaning on your left arm.

- Keep your ankle stabilized and bend your right knee.

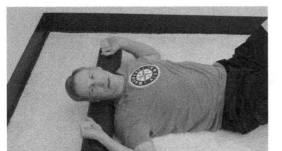

NECK

- Rolling your neck is very simple and feels great. Lying flat on your back, place the roller underneath your neck. The roller will be as close to your shoulders as possible.

- Close your eyes and just relax, taking deep breaths.

- Roll your head to the right and then to the left. Pausing at any tender areas along the way.

HIP FLEXOR, GLUTES, HAMSTRING

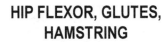

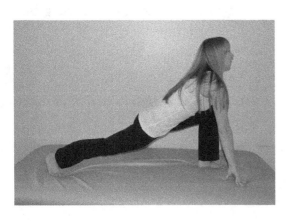

- Standing with your feet together, place one leg forward into a lunge position.

- Keeping your back leg straight and your forward knee above your heel, lean forward at the hips and place both hands on the ground.

- Move your weight down toward the ground.

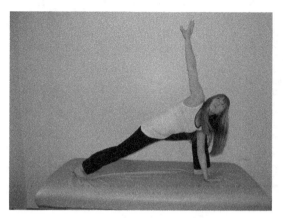

HIP FLEXOR, GLUTES, HAMSTRING, LOWER BACK

- Place your left leg forward into a lunge position.
- Keeping your right leg straight and your left knee above your heel, lean forward at the hips and place your left hand on the inside of your left foot.
- Pushing your left elbow into your knee, turn your body, and reach to the sky with your right arm.

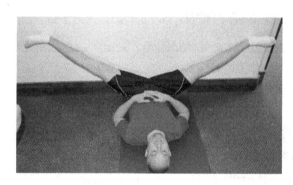

ADDUCTORS, HAMSTRINGS, LOWER BACK

- Lie on your back on the floor, pulling yourself in toward the wall. Straighten your legs up the wall.
- Slowly lower your legs out to the side.

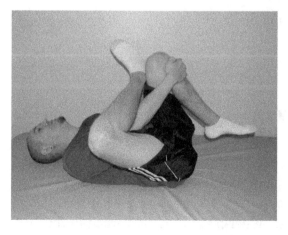

GLUTES

- Lie on your back with both knees bent.
- Place your right ankle on your left knee.
- Take your right arm through your legs and grasp your knee. Take your left hand and place it on your right hand, interlocking your fingers.
- Pull your left knee toward your chest, feeling this stretch in your right hip.

UPPER BACK

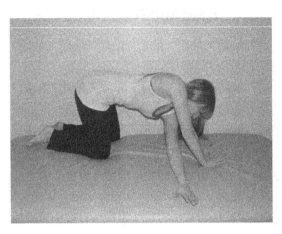

- Start this stretch from your hands and knees.
- Keeping one arm straight, slide your other arm under your body and lower your shoulder to the ground. Reach with the arm on the floor.
- Relax and hold the stretch, ensuring proper breathing.
- Placing your palm down will intensify the stretch.

CHEST AND FRONT OF SHOULDERS

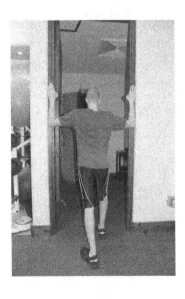

- Start by standing in a doorway. Bend your elbows to a 90-degree angle.
- Place your hands and elbows on each side of the doorway. I try to keep my elbows up at shoulder height. Changing the height will change the angle of the stretch.
- Place one leg forward through the doorway.
- Keeping your posture nice and tall, slowly lean your body forward into the stretch.
- Relax and hold the stretch, ensuring proper breathing.

MY FAVORITE STRETCHES (PROGRAM #3)

The stretches in this program are some of my favorites because of some of my problems that I have dealt with in the past. I put all of these together simply because I love all of these stretches and they have a great impact on your body and target areas that people typically don't work on by themselves. Areas like your rotator cuff, foot, hip flexors, and muscles between your shoulder blades are all worked in this well rounded program.

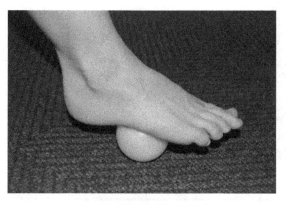

- Although this is not a foam roller, using a medium-size ball is a wonderful way to stretch and massage the muscles and tendons on the bottom of your foot. This is a great therapeutic exercise for plantar fascia and other issues causing foot pain. The use of different size balls will change the intensity of pressure on your foot. Move slowly onto the ball, making sure to not to place your entire body weight on top.

HIP FLEXOR

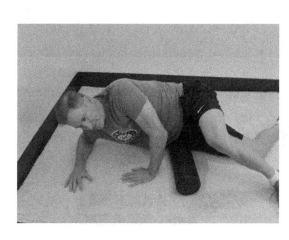

- Place the roller on the group of muscles just under your hip bone.
- If you are working on your left side, your left leg will be straight. Bend your right leg at a 90-degree angle and place your right foot on the ground.
- While resting on your left elbow, your right hand will be on the floor, giving you more balance.
- Lean slightly to the left side and do short movements up and down your hip flexor muscles.

HAMSTRING

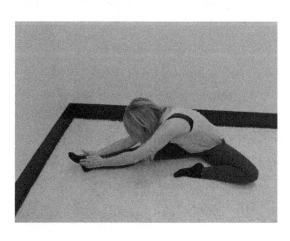

- In a seated position, straighten one leg and place it out into a splits position. Bend your other leg and bring your foot in close to your body.
- Keeping your posture nice and tall, bend toward the straightened leg.
- Relax and hold the stretch, ensuring proper breathing.

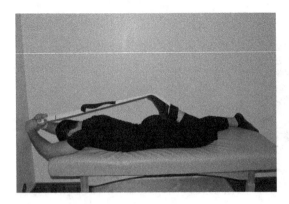

THIGH, SHIN, TOP OF FOOT

- Place a TStretch strap around your foot and lie flat on your stomach.
- Holding the strap with both hands, begin to pull your foot up toward your rear end.
- Relax and hold the stretch, ensuring proper breathing.

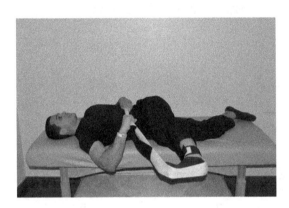

HAMSTRING, HIP, AND LOWER BACK

- Place a TStretch strap around your left foot and lie on your right side.
- Holding the strap, keep your left leg straight.
- Slowly push your left shoulder back on the floor/ bed and pull your left leg up toward your head.

ADDUCTORS AND LOWER BACK

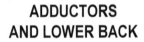
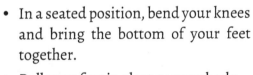

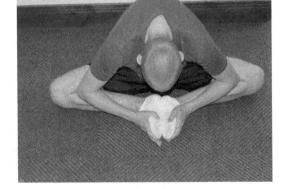

- In a seated position, bend your knees and bring the bottom of your feet together.
- Pull your feet in close to your body.
- Let your knees lay down to the ground. Pushing your knees down with your elbows, slowly lean forward.
- Relax and hold position, ensuring proper breathing.

UPPER AND LOWER BACK

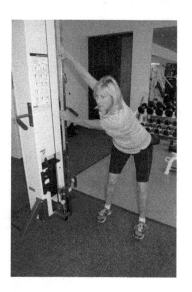

- Begin by standing with your side approximately one foot away from a door jamb or a secure post.

- With your feet shoulder width apart, grasp a door jamb or secure post with both hands (thumbs should point towards each other).

- Place the closest hand on the top about head height and the lower hand even with the lower portion of your chest.

- Making sure your hips are pointed forward, pull with your lower arm, and push with your upper arm.

- Relax and hold the stretch, ensuring proper breathing.

ROTATOR CUFF

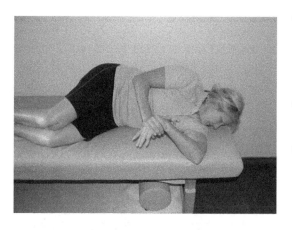

- Lying on your side, bring your arm out to a 90-degree angle. Bend your elbow and wrist also to a 90-degree angle.

- Looking straight down, place your chin on your shoulder.

- Using your other hand, grab your wrist and gently push your elbow down into the ground. Slowly push your hand down toward the floor.

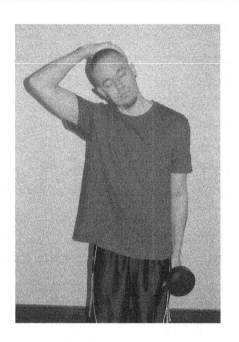

SIDE OF NECK

- In a standing position, hold a weight or some sort of stationary object like a table. The idea is to keep your shoulder down.
- With the other hand, slowly pull the side of your head toward the floor.
- Relax and hold the stretch, ensuring proper breathing.

BEGINNER STRETCHING ROUTINE

This routine contains a number of stretches that I feel are important not just for beginners, but for anyone looking to improve their flexibility and overall wellbeing. Within this routine, I give you stretches for your hamstrings, hip flexors, groin, glutes, back, chest, and triceps (back of arms).

HAMSTRING

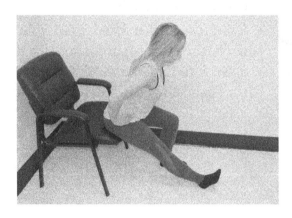

- Sit toward the end of a chair with one leg bent and the other leg straight out with the heel on the floor.
- Keeping your posture nice and tall, bend forward at the hips until you reach a stretched position. Do not hunch your back.
- Relax and hold the stretch, ensuring proper breathing.

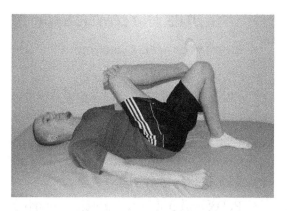

GLUTES AND LOWER BACK

- Lie on your back with both knees bent.
- Place your right ankle on your left knee.
- Using your left hand, grasp your right knee and pull your knee down toward your chest.
- Relax and hold the stretch, ensuring proper breathing.

ADDUCTORS

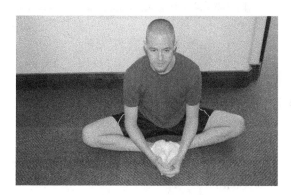

- In a seated position, bend your knees and bring the bottom of your feet together.
- Sitting nice and tall, pull your feet in close to your body.
- Let your knees lay down to the ground.
- Relax and hold the position, ensuring proper breathing.

HIP FLEXOR

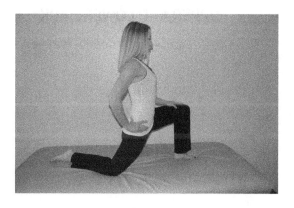

- Get down on both knees and place one foot forward in a lunge position.
- Take your weight down and forward, keeping your posture nice and tall.
- Relax and hold the stretch, ensuring proper breathing.

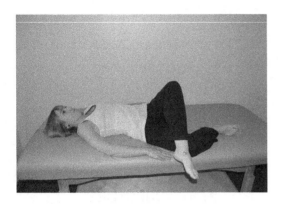

GLUTES AND LOWER BACK

- Lie on your back, place your left ankle on your right knee.
- Pull your right foot in and lay the outside of your right knee down on the floor.
- Continue to pull your right knee and foot in until you feel a stretch.
- Relax and hold the stretch, ensuring proper breathing.

LOWER BACK

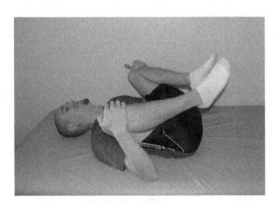

- Lie on your back.
- Pull both knees up toward your chest.
- Grasping your knees with your hands, pull your knees in toward your chest and out away from each other.
- Relax and hold the stretch, ensuring proper breathing.

UPPER AND LOWER BACK

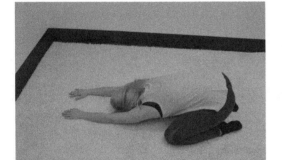

- On your hands and knees, lower your rear end to your heels.
- Reach your hands out above your head and push your chest to the floor.
- Relax and hold the stretch, ensuring proper breathing.

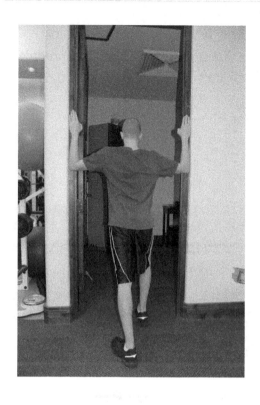

CHEST AND FRONT OF SHOULDERS

- Start by standing in a doorway. Bend your elbows to a 90-degree angle.
- Place your hands and elbows on each side of the doorway. I try to keep my elbows up at shoulder height. Changing the height will change the angle of the stretch.
- Place one leg forward through the doorway.
- Keeping your posture nice and tall, slowly lean your body forward into the stretch.
- Relax and hold the stretch, ensuring proper breathing.

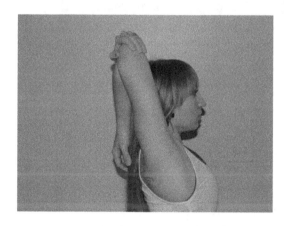

BACK OF ARM

- In a standing or seated position, raise your arm over your head, bending at your elbow.
- Take your other hand and grab your elbow.
- Slowly pull your elbow back behind your head.
- Relax and hold the stretch, ensuring proper breathing.

INTERMEDIATE STRETCHING ROUTINE

The intermediate routine I wanted to add in a little bit of the foam roller and continue to work on some of those same muscle groups in the beginner routine, but in a more complex way. Within this program, we will work on the IT band, hamstrings, glutes, adductors, thighs, hip flexors, shoulders, chest, and neck.

IT BAND

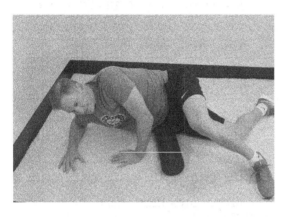

- Start by laying the outside of your leg on the roller. In the beginning position, the leg on the roller should remain straight while the other leg is bent and the foot is resting on the ground.
- Once you feel comfortable, slowly roll lengthwise up and down. Find those tender areas and hold for 15-30 seconds.

GLUTES

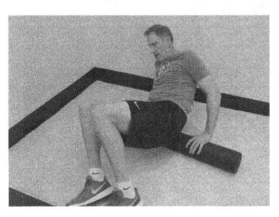

- Sit on the foam roller with your hands on the ground behind you.
- Bend both knees, keeping knees and feet together.
- Rotate your knees to the side, stabilizing yourself with the one arm that you are leaning toward. Slowly roll the muscles in your hips.

HAMSTRING

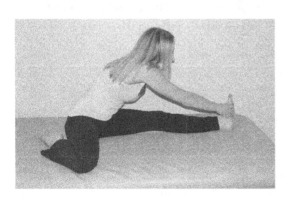

- In a seated position, place one leg straight out in front of you. Bend the other leg and place the foot behind you with your knee pointed out.
- Keeping your posture nice and tall, bend forward at the hips.
- Slowly reach for your toes.

GLUTES

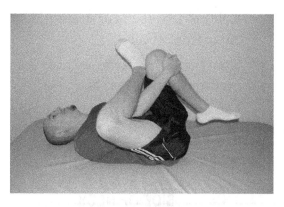

- Lie on your back with both knees bent.
- Place your right ankle on your left knee.
- Take your right arm through your legs and grasp your knee. Take your left hand and place it on your right hand, interlocking your fingers.
- Pull your left knee toward your chest, feeling this stretch in your right hip.

ADDUCTORS

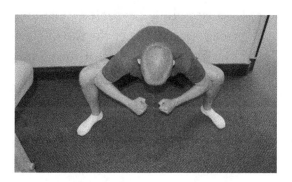

- Stand with your feet approximately three feet apart.
- Squat down, keeping your knees above your heels.
- Place your elbows on the inside of your knees and push out.

THIGH AND HIP FLEXOR

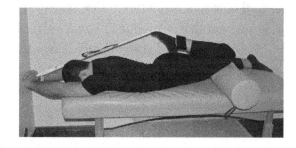

- Lying on your stomach, place a riser like a pillow or the foam roller just above your knee.
- Place the strap around your foot and pull your foot toward your head.

FRONT OF SHOULDER AND BICEPS

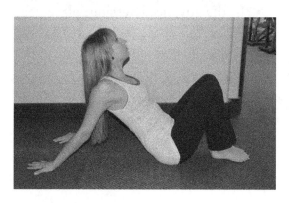

- In a seated position, bend your knees and place your arms behind you.
- Slightly raise your rear end off the ground and slowly move toward your feet until you feel a stretch.
- Lower your rear end to the floor, keeping your back straight. Don't let your chest sink down.

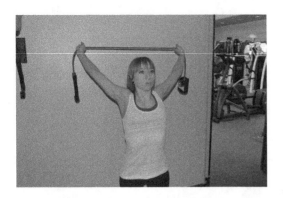

CHEST AND FRONT OF SHOULDERS

- Hold an elastic band or strap straight out in front of you.
- Slowly raise your arms up over your head and behind your back.
- Relax and hold the stretch, ensuring proper breathing.

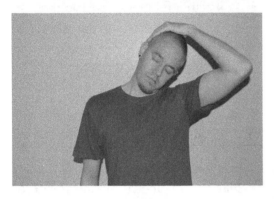

SIDE OF NECK

- In a standing or seated position, place your hand over the top of your head, grabbing the side of your head.
- Slowly pull your head to the side.
- Relax and hold the stretch, ensuring proper breathing.

ADVANCED STRETCHING ROUTINE

The advanced routine focuses on the individual who has more flexibility, strength, and balance. I have given you a well rounded program that hits your IT band, calves, hamstrings, adductors, thighs, hip flexors, glutes, back, and upper body. I would recommend this program for individuals that are more experienced with their stretching.

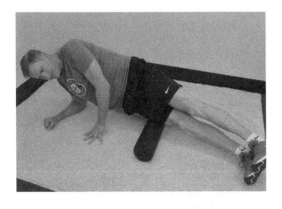

IT BAND

- In the advanced version, place your leg on top of the leg you are rolling. This will allow your own body to put more weight on the roller.
- Once you feel comfortable, slowly roll lengthwise up and down. Find those tender areas and hold for 15-30 seconds.

GLUTES AND PIRIFORMIS

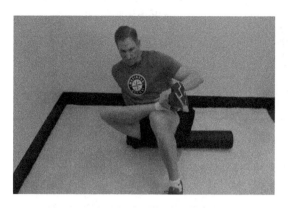

- Start by placing your right ankle on your straightened left leg, just above the knee. Ensure you are leaning on your right arm.
- Keep your ankle stabilized and bend your left knee.
- Slowly roll up and down your hip. Take note that you are now rolling a muscle that is actually getting stretched at the same time. This will be a very tender area when you first begin.

CALVES

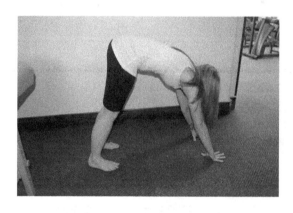

- Begin this stretch in a push up position.
- Slowly move your hands back toward your feet and lift your hips higher in the air.
- Slowly push your heels back into the ground.
- Relax and hold the stretch, ensuring proper breathing.
- End the stretch by returning to a push up position.

HAMSTRING

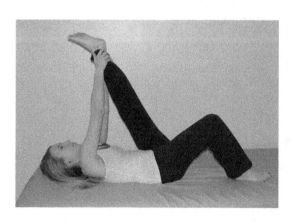

- Lie on your back, bend one knee so the bottom of your foot rests flat on the floor.
- Raise the other leg off the floor and grasp the lower portion of your calf.
- Keep your leg straight while pulling it towards you.
- Relax and hold the stretch, ensuring proper breathing.

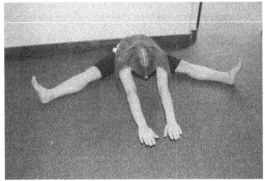

ADDUCTORS, HAMSTRINGS, LOWER BACK

- In a seated position, spread your legs as far as they will go.
- Keeping your posture nice and tall and your toes pointed up, bend forward at the hips.
- Relax and hold the stretch, ensuring proper breathing.

ADDUCTORS

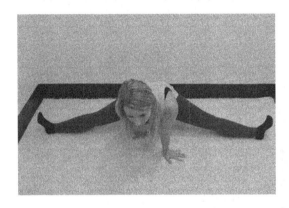

- In a standing position, slowly spread your feet apart.
- Ensuring your toes are pointed up, lower your body as far as you can (into a full split if you are able). Balance yourself by placing your hands on the floor or other stable object.
- Relax and hold the stretch, ensuring proper breathing.

HIP FLEXOR, GLUTES, HAMSTRING, LOWER BACK

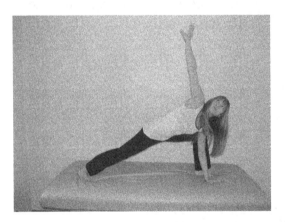

- Place your left leg forward into a lunge position.
- Keeping your right leg straight and your left knee above your heel, lean forward at the hips and place your left hand on the inside of your left foot.
- Pushing your left elbow into your knee, turn your body, and reach to the sky with your right arm.

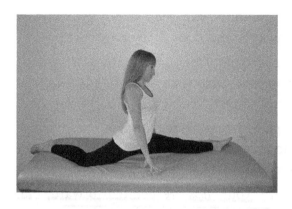

HAMSTRING AND HIP FLEXOR

- Standing with your feet together, place one leg forward, and slowly begin to slide your feet further apart.
- Keeping your posture nice and tall, move down into a slide split position. Stabilize yourself with your hands if needed.
- Relax and hold the position, ensuring proper breathing.

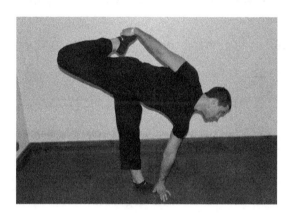

HIP FLEXOR, THIGH, HAMSTRING

- In a standing position, grab a foot and pull it up to your rear end.
- Keeping hold of your foot, slowly lean forward and touch your hand to the floor.
- Keep your posture nice and tall.
- Relax and hold the position, ensuring proper breathing.

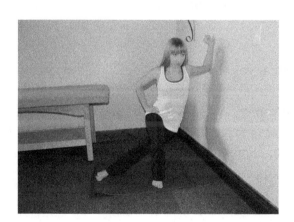

HIP AND IT BAND

- Stand approximately elbow length away from the wall.
- Take the leg closest to the wall and cross it behind you. Slide it away from the wall as you slowly lower down toward the ground. Do not let your forward knee get past your toes.

UPPER AND LOWER BACK

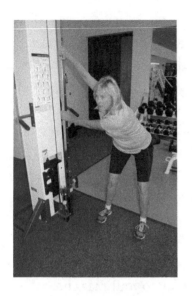

- Begin by standing with your side approximately one foot away from a door jamb or a secure post.
- With your feet shoulder width apart, grasp a door jamb or secure post with both hands (thumbs should point towards each other).
- Place the closest hand on the top about head height and the lower hand even with the lower portion of your chest.
- Making sure your hips are pointed forward, pull with your lower arm, and push with your upper arm.
- Relax and hold the stretch, ensuring proper breathing.

SHOULDERS AND BACK OF ARMS

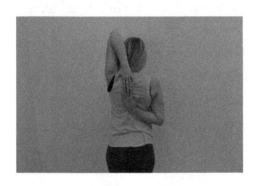

- Place one arm behind your back, and one arm bent over your head.
- Interlock your fingers and slowly pull your hands together.
- Relax and hold the stretch, ensuring proper breathing.

PARTNER ASSISTED ROUTINE

If you are lucky enough to have a partner that you fully trust, I would highly suggest you do this routine! Partner assisted stretching is my favorite form due to your ability to totally relax your entire body while someone else is helping you do the work so you can relax and focus on the area being stretched. I do, however, stress the importance of taking this seriously and not allowing your partner to push you past your limits. Communicate all the time, letting your partner know how much further you can go, or if it is too much. I also love this program because most of your body is getting stretched.

HAMSTRING

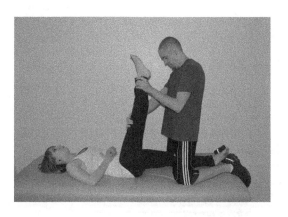

- While lying on your back, have your partner pick one leg up, placing one hand just above the knee on your thigh and the other hand just above your heel.

- Keeping your leg straight, have your partner slowly push your leg back until the stretch is felt.

- Relax and hold the stretch, ensuring proper breathing.

GLUTES

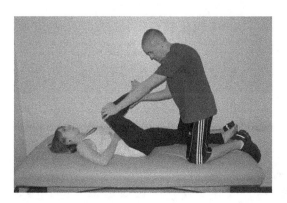

- Lying on your back, have your partner take hold of your leg, placing one hand on the side of your knee and the other hand on your ankle.

- Keeping your leg at a 90-degree angle, have your partner GENTLY push your knee toward your chest.

ADDUCTORS

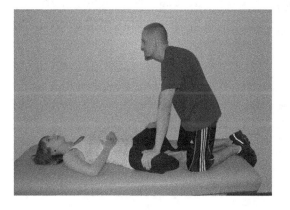

- Lying on your back, place the bottom of your feet together and relax your knees out.

- Have your partner GENTLY push your knees down toward the table.

- Relax and hold the stretch, ensuring proper breathing.

- Communicate with your partner, letting him/her know when you feel the stretch.

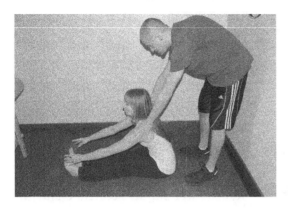

HAMSTRINGS

- Sit with your legs straight out in front of you.
- Keeping your posture nice and tall, have your partner GENTLY push on your upper back, reaching for your toes.
- Relax and hold the stretch, ensuring proper breathing.
- Communicate with your partner, letting him/her know when you feel the stretch.

ADDUCTORS, HAMSTRINGS, LOWER BACK

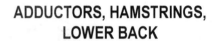

- In a seated position, spread your legs as far out as they can go.
- Keeping your posture tall, have your partner GENTLY push down on your upper back.
- Relax and hold the stretch, ensuring proper breathing.
- Communicate with your partner, letting him/her know when you feel the stretch.

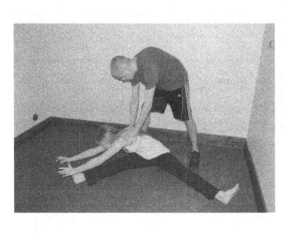

- In a seated position, spread your legs as far out as they will go.
- While trying to avoid hunching over, reach down toward your foot. Have your partner GENTLY push down on your upper back.
- Relax and hold the stretch, ensuring proper breathing.

HIP FLEXOR

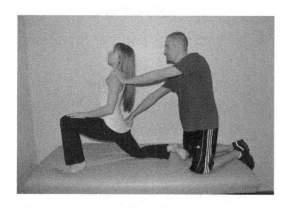

- Get down on both knees and place one foot out into a lunge position. Keeping your posture tall, move your body forward and hips down toward the floor.

- Have your partner place his/her fist just above your glutes and have them push down and forward.

- Relax and hold the stretch, ensuring proper breathing.

HIP FLEXOR AND THIGH

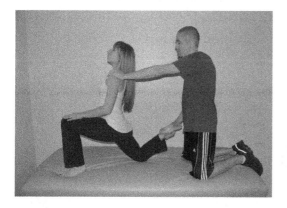

- Get down on both knees and place one foot out into a lunge position. Keeping your posture tall, move your body forward and hips down toward the floor.

- Have your partner grab the top of your foot and GENTLY pull your foot up off the ground.

- Relax and hold the stretch, ensuring proper breathing.

CHEST AND FRONT OF SHOULDERS

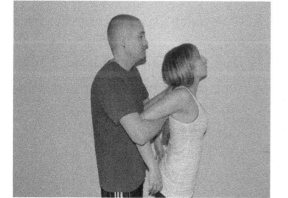

- In a standing position, have your partner hold underneath your bent arms with their hands on your back.

- Keeping your posture nice and tall, have your partner slowly squeeze your arms together.

- Relax and hold the stretch, ensuring proper breathing.

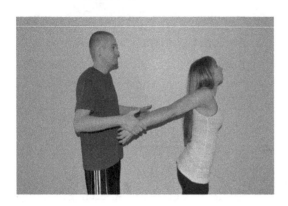

CHEST, FRONT OF SHOULDERS, AND BICEPS

- In a standing position, have your partner hold your wrists with your arms straight behind you.
- Keeping your posture nice and tall, have your partner slowly raise and squeeze your arms together.
- Relax and hold the stretch, ensuring proper breathing.

CHEST

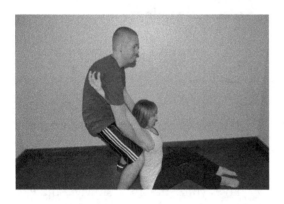

- In a seated position on the floor, interlock your hands and place them behind your head.
- Your partner will place his/her forearms over your arms and place their hands on your back.
- Have your partner slowly pull back on your arms while pushing forward on your back.

- Reach your arms above your head from a seated position on the floor.
- Have your partner place his/her arms over yours and place their hands on your back, over your shoulder blades.
- Your partner will slowly lean back while pushing your back forward.

LATS AND RIBS

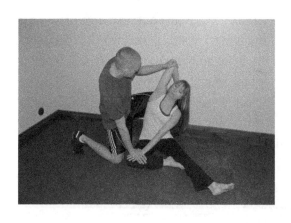

- Sitting on the ground, place your left leg straight out in front of you with your right leg bent and the bottom of your right foot against your left leg.

- Place your right hand on the back of your head with your left hand on your right knee.

- Have your partner kneel down with his/her left knee pushing slightly against your back.

- Your partner will place his/her right hand on the hand that is on your knee and his/her left hand on your elbow.

- Have your partner slowly push your elbow, causing you to lean to the side while pushing down on your knee.

- Relax and hold the stretch, ensuring proper breathing.

- Repeat on the other side.

NECK

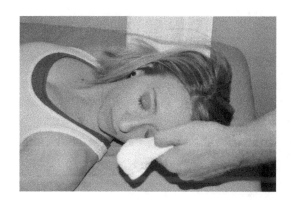

- Lying on your back, center a hand towel, folded lengthwise, under your head.

- Your partner will grab the towel on both ends and slightly raise your head off the table or floor.

- Your partner will then slowly raise one end of the towel, turning your head to the side.

STRAP STRETCHING ROUTINE

Using a strap is a form of passive stretching that utilizes an outside force to assist you with a stretch. Utilizing the strap will allow you to stretch muscles that you normally wouldn't be able to stretch on your own. This routine can be utilized by anybody but is particularly beneficial for individuals that are a little tighter and need help getting into certain positions. I would highly suggest a strap to anyone, you may find that you truly enjoy the stretch it provides your muscles. This program contains stretches for your calf, hamstrings, adductors, glutes, lower back, chest, shoulders, and triceps.

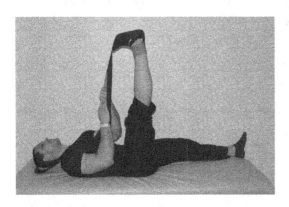

CALF

- Lying flat on your back, place the TStretch strap around your ankle and up the bottom of your foot.
- Bring your leg straight up and pull back and down on the strap.

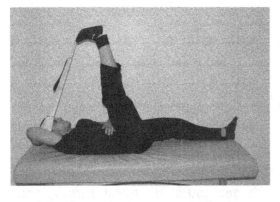

LOWER HAMSTRING

- Lying on your back, place the TStretch strap around your ankle and up the bottom of your foot.
- Keeping your leg straight, pull your leg towards you.

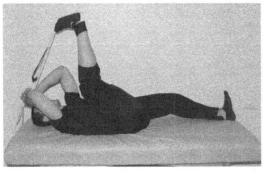

UPPER HAMSTRING

- Lying on your back, place the TStretch strap around your ankle and under the bottom of your foot.
- With your knee bent, pull leg down and toward your head.

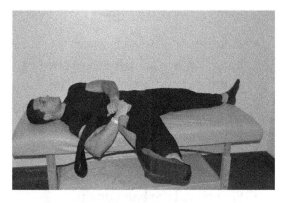

ADDUCTOR

- Place a TStretch strap around your foot and lie flat on your back.
- Take your leg as far out to the side as you can.
- Using one arm, pull on the strap, pulling your leg out even further.

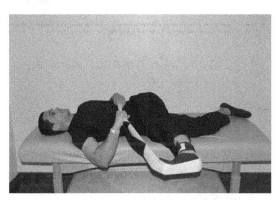

GLUTES AND LOWER BACK

- Place a TStretch strap around your left foot and lie on your right side.
- Holding the strap, keep your left leg straight.
- Slowly push your left shoulder back on the floor/ bed and pull your left leg up toward your head.

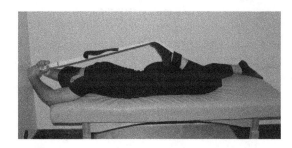

THIGH

- Place a TStretch strap around your foot and lie flat on your stomach.
- Holding the strap with both hands, begin to pull your foot up toward your rear end.

HIP FLEXOR AND THIGH

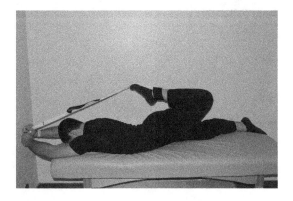

- Place a TStretch strap around your ankle and up over your toes.
- Lie on your stomach, holding the strap behind your head.
- Pull the strap over your head, lifting your knee off the ground.

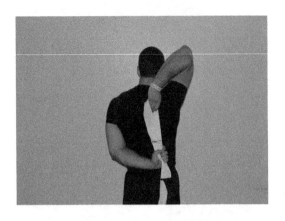

TRICEP

- Holding a TStretch strap in your hand, raise your arm over your head and bend it at your elbow. The strap should be hanging straight down behind your back.
- Grab the strap with your other hand behind your back.
- Slowly pull the band down.

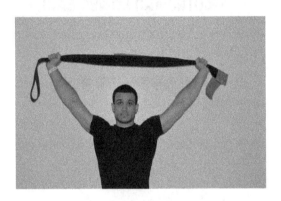

CHEST

- Hold an elastic band or strap straight out in front of you.
- Slowly raise your arms up over your head and behind your back.
- Always start with your hands further apart and move them in if you have to.

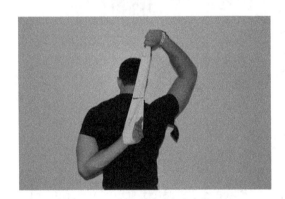

SHOULDER

- Place your arm behind your back.
- Place your other arm over your head with your elbow bent, holding a strap in your hand.
- Grab hold of the strap behind your back and slowly pull your arm up your back.

LOWER BACK STRETCHING ROUTINE (SCARED TO BEND OVER ROUTINE)

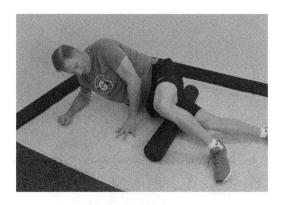

IT BAND

- Start by laying the outside of your leg on the roller. In the beginning position, the leg on the roller should remain straight while the other leg is bent and the foot is resting on the ground.

- Once you feel comfortable, slowly roll lengthwise up and down. Find those tender areas and hold for 15-30 seconds.

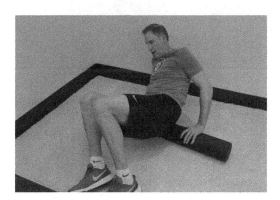

GLUTES

- Sit on the foam roller with your hands on the ground behind you.

- Bend both knees, keeping knees and feet together.

- Rotate your knees to the side, stabilizing yourself with the one arm that you are leaning toward. Slowly roll the muscles in your hips.

HIP FLEXOR

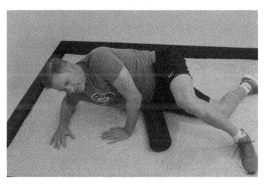

- Place the roller on the group of muscles just under your hip bone.

- If you are working on your left side, your left leg will be straight. Bend your right leg at a 90-degree angle and place your right foot on the ground. This position will give you a better base in which to move.

- While resting on your left elbow, your right hand will be on the floor, giving you more balance.

- Lean slightly to the left side and do short movements up and down your hip flexor muscles.

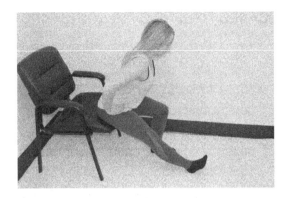

HAMSTRING

- Sit toward the end of a chair with one leg bent and the other leg straight out with the heel on the floor.
- Keeping your posture nice and tall, bend forward at the hips until you reach a stretched position. Do not hunch your back.

GLUTES

- In a seated position, place your right ankle on your left knee.
- Sitting in a nice and tall position, slowly push your knee down.

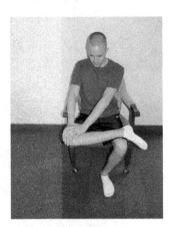

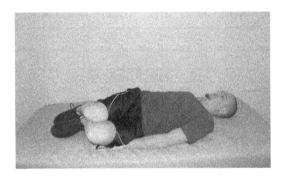

- Lying on your back, bend your knees and place your feet flat on the floor/bed.
- Slowly move your knees to the side, keeping them together until you feel the stretch.
- Return to the starting position and repeat on the other side. Repeat 15-20 times.

ADDUCTORS

- Lying on your back, bend your knees and place your feet flat on the floor/bed.
- Slowly spread your knees apart from each other until the stretch is felt.
- Return to the starting position and repeat the stretch. Repeat 15-20 times.

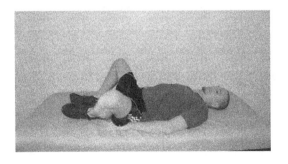

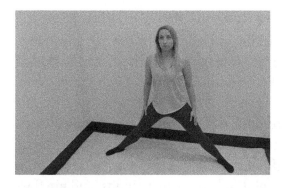

- In a standing position, slowly spread your feet apart until you feel the stretch in between your legs.
- Keep your posture nice and tall.
- Relax and hold the position, ensuring proper breathing.

HIP FLEXOR

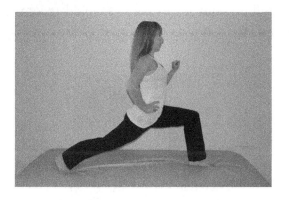

- Standing with your feet together, place one leg forward into a lunge position.
- Keeping your back leg straight and your forward knee above your heel, move your weight down toward the ground. Ensure your posture is nice and tall.

ABDOMINALS

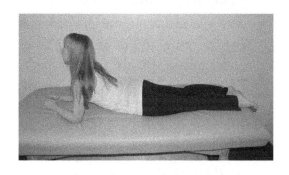

- Lie on your stomach.
- Place your elbows underneath your shoulders and rise up. Look straight ahead.
- Relax and hold the stretch, ensuring proper breathing.

BACK

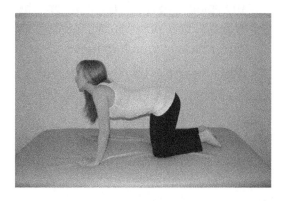

- Get on your hands and knees.
- Breathing out, let your chest and stomach sink down to the ground as you raise your head up.
- Relax and hold the stretch, ensuring proper breathing.
- Combine this stretch with the stretch below for a great functional movement for the spine.

LOWER BACK STRETCHING ROUTINE (NO RESTRICTION ROUTINE)

I have been working with in the field of "flexibility therapy" for over 20 years now, and I can tell you that the one thing you never want to deal with is a bad back! For those of you that have had the issue, I feel your pain; for those of you that haven't, good for you and do whatever you can to stay away. Regardless of where you fit, this is a great routine to help you stay away from those debilitating back pains. What I want to get across in this routine is the fact that your lower body has a great impact on back pain. You will notice that most of the stretches in this routine aren't even back stretches, but stretches more for your glutes, hamstrings, thighs, and hip flexors. When those muscles get tight, they pull on your lower back. I would recommend everyone do this routine, just take note that some of the stretches are a little more advanced.

IT BAND

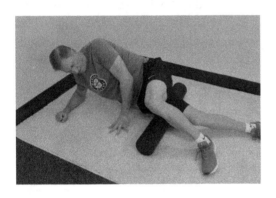

- Start by laying the outside of your leg on the roller. The leg on the roller should remain straight while the other leg is bent, and the foot is resting on the ground.
- Once you feel comfortable, slowly roll lengthwise up and down. Find those tender areas and hold for 15-30 seconds.

HIP FLEXOR

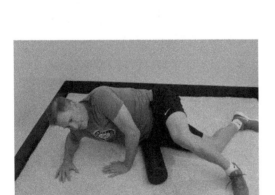

- If you are working on your left side, your left leg will be straight. Bend your right leg at a 90-degree angle and place your right foot on the ground. This position will give you a better base in which to move.
- While resting on your left elbow, your right hand will be on the floor, giving you more balance.
- Lean slightly to the left side and do short movements up and down your hip flexor muscles.

- This action is great for helping lower back pain. Our hip flexors attach in the front portion of our body, go through the hip and attach in the lower back. These muscles are a major cause of the inability to stand up straight after sitting for a long period of time.

BACK

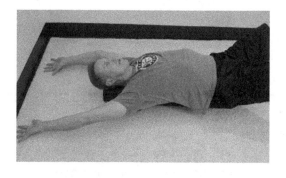

- Lie on the roller lengthwise with your head, upper back, and tailbone supported. Bend both knees and keep your feet flat on the floor for support.
- Draw your navel in and perform a pelvic tilt, laying your lower back on the roller.

- To add a little extra pressure to your upper back, bring your arms straight up above your head. Keep your lower back against the roller and relax.

HAMSTRING

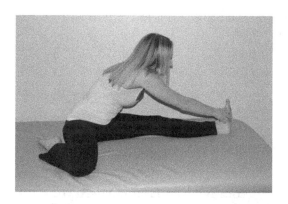

- In a seated position, place one leg straight out in front of you. Bend the other leg and place the foot behind you with your knee pointed out.
- Keeping your posture nice and tall, bend forward at the hips.
- Slowly reach for your toes.

ADDUCTORS AND HAMSTRINGS

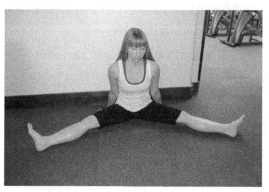

- Start in a seated position, keeping your posture nice and tall.
- Spread your legs as far as they will let you go.
- If you have a tendency to want to lean back, sit with your back against a wall to keep you from rocking back.

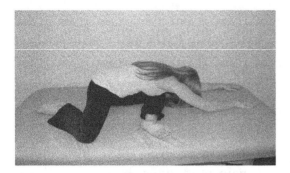

GLUTES

- In a seated position, bend one leg and place it behind you and bend your forward leg to a 90-degree angle.

- Keeping your posture nice and tall, lean forward toward your knee.

HIP FLEXOR, GLUTES, LOWER BACK, HAMSTRING

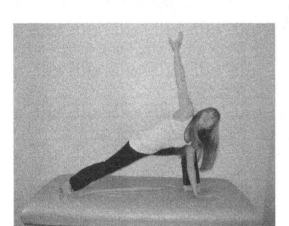

- Place your left leg forward into a lunge position.

- Keeping your right leg straight and your left knee above your heel, lean forward at the hips and place your left hand on the inside of your left foot.

- Pushing your left elbow into your knee, turn your body, and reach to the sky with your right arm.

THIGH AND HIP FLEXOR

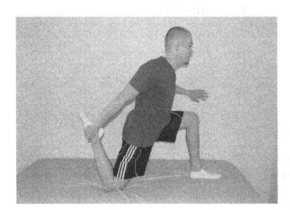

- Get down on both knees and place one foot forward in a lunge position.

- Reach behind you and take ahold of your foot. Pull it up toward your hip. If needed, hold on to a stable object to help with balance.

- Take your weight down and forward, keeping your posture nice and tall.

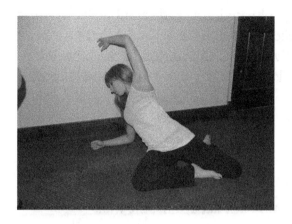

HIPS AND LOWER BACK

- From a seated position, bend one knee and place it behind you. Bend your opposite knee and place your foot against your leg.
- Keeping your posture tall, rotate your body toward your front leg and place your back elbow on the floor.
- Keeping your chest up, reach your forward arm over your head, extending your arm.

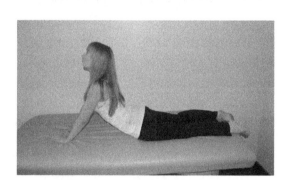

ABDOMINALS

- Lie on your stomach.
- Place your hands underneath your shoulders and rise up. Look straight ahead.
- Relax and hold the stretch, ensuring proper breathing.

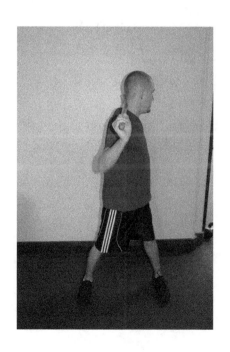

LOWER BACK AND CHEST (IF TIGHT)

- Stand with your feet approximately shoulder-width apart.
- Carefully place and hold a pole of some sort on your upper back and shoulders.
- Keeping your posture nice and tall, rotate your upper body to the side.

ARTHRITIC HIP PAIN STRETCHING ROUTINE

Arthritis can cause a tremendous amount of pain in the body and I do believe that stretching can help ease the pain. The following routine is a routine that I have had good luck with when working with individuals with arthritis in the hips. Please understand that not all of these may work for you, but give it a shot and stick with the stretches that help you. The goal is to loosen up any of those muscles that may be causing your hip joint to tighten up. In turn, we hope to create a little more space in that joint so you don't have so much bone on bone friction.

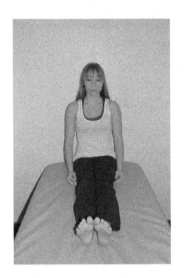

HAMSTRINGS AND LOWER BACK

- Sit with your back flat against the wall.
- Place your legs together, straight out in front of you.
- Keeping your posture nice and tall, move your rear end toward the wall.

GLUTES

- Lie on your back.
- Place your right ankle on your left knee.
- Rest your knee down to the table.

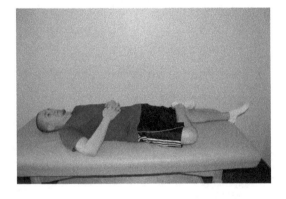

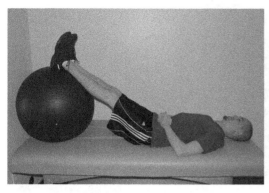 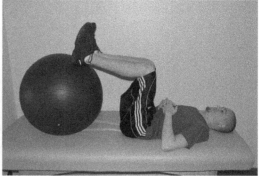

HAMSTRINGS AND GLUTES

- Lying on your back, place your heels near the center of a therapy ball.
- Bending your knees, slowly pull the ball in toward your rear end until you feel the stretch.
- Move the ball back to the starting position and repeat. Repeat 15-20 times.

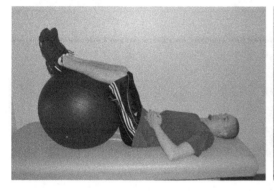 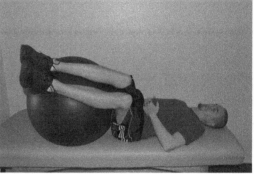

HIPS AND LOWER BACK

- Lying on your back, place your legs on top of a therapy ball.
- Slowly rotate the ball to the side until you feel the stretch.
- Move back to the starting position and repeat the stretch to the other side. Repeat 15-20 times.

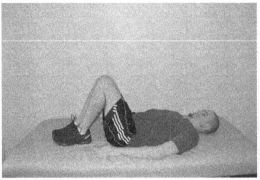 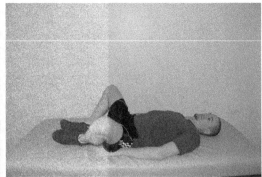

ADDUCTORS

- Lying on your back, bend your knees and place your **feet flat on the floor/bed.**
- Slowly spread your knees apart from each other until the stretch is felt.
- Return to the starting position and repeat the stretch. **Repeat 15-20 times.**

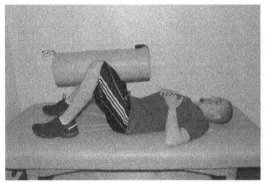 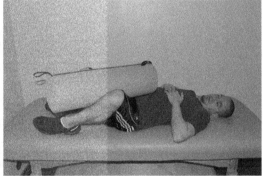

HIPS AND LOWER BACK

- Lying on your back, bend your knees and place your **feet flat on the floor/bed.**
- Place something between your knees like a pillow or ball. Squeezing the object, slowly move your knees to the side until you feel the **stretch.**
- Return to the starting position and repeat on the other side. Repeat 15-20 times.

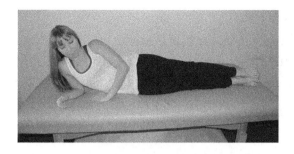

- Lie on your side with your legs together.
- Prop yourself up on your elbow, placing the elbow under your shoulder.
- Support yourself with your other arm.

ADDUCTORS

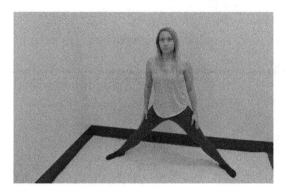

- In a standing position, slowly spread your feet apart until you feel the stretch in between your legs.
- Keep your posture nice and tall.

HIP FLEXOR

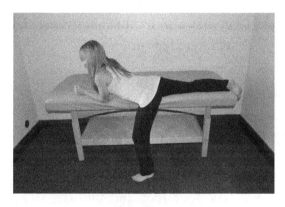

- Using your bed or table, lie on your stomach on the side of the table with one leg supporting you on the ground.
- Put your elbows underneath your shoulders and rise up, looking straight ahead. Focus on pushing your thigh into the table.

HIP AND LOWER BACK

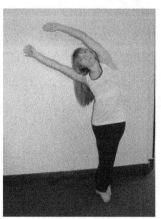

- Stand with your feet together and your posture nice and tall.
- Cross one leg in front of the other.
- Raise your arms high above your head and lean to the side where your foot is crossed.
- Keep your posture nice and tall and pointed forward. Try not to turn your body. Reach as high as you can.

KNEE REPLACEMENT STRETCHING ROUTINE

If you have had a knee replacement and you are looking at this routine, I hope you understand the importance of keeping your knee moving. As you are aware, not only being able to bend your knee, but also being able to straighten it is imperative. The following stretches were added to assist you in keeping your knee moving AFTER you have finished your physical therapy. As always check with your doctor before starting any new program.

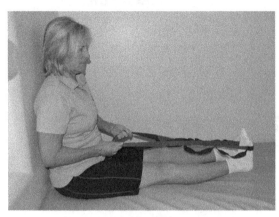

- Sit with both legs straight in front of you.
- Place a strap or towel around the ball of your foot (just below your toes).
- Relax your foot and pull the strap back.
- Relax and hold the stretch, ensuring proper breathing.
- You may also want to sit against the wall for added support.

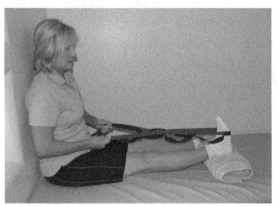

- Sitting with both legs straight in front of you, place a rolled-up towel under your heel.
- Place a strap or towel around the ball of your foot (just below your toes).
- Relax your foot and pull the strap back.
- Relax and hold the stretch, ensuring proper breathing.
- Sitting against the wall will give you some added support.

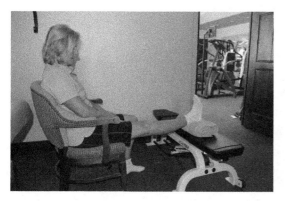

- Sit in a chair with another chair or stationary object in front of you. Place a rolled-up towel on the chair in front of you.
- Put your foot on top of the towel and relax your knee down toward the ground.
- Relax and hold the stretch, ensuring proper breathing.

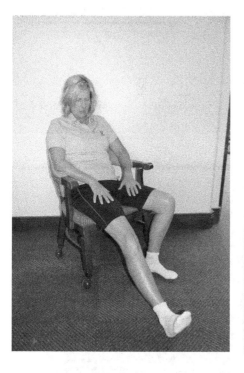 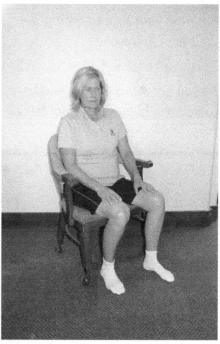

- Sitting in a chair, start with your leg straightened.
- Keeping your posture tall, slowly move your heel in under the chair.

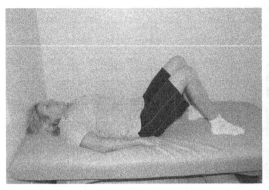 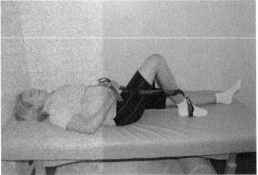

- Lie on the floor/bed with both legs in a straightened position.
- Keeping your foot touching the floor or bed, slowly bend your knee, bringing your heel in toward your glutes.
- Relax and hold the stretch, ensuring proper breathing.
- As you get more movement in your knee, you can also begin to use a strap or towel to help pull your foot back.

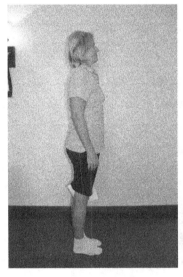 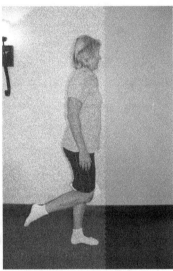

- In a standing position, place a towel between your knees.
- Squeezing the towel, slowly bend your knee, bringing your foot up behind you.
- Don't let the towel fall.
- Relax and hold the stretch, ensuring proper breathing.
- Hold on to the wall or other stationary object for stability.

PLANTAR FASCIA STRETCHING ROUTINE

I joke around with my clients telling them that I feel that I always have to get what they have so I can help understand what they are feeling. I have suffered from plantar fasciitis before and it can be unbelievably painful. It has taken me off my feet so I couldn't stand before. The following routine is all about trying to loosen all of the muscles in the feet, ankles, calves, and even hamstrings. Try this routine, but I also want you to look at your diet as well. I have had a couple clients that have changed their diet and their pain went away. Try to avoid anything acidic for a while such as sodas, alcohol, red meat, and sugar.

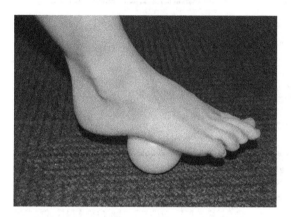

- Although this is not a foam roller, using a medium-size ball is a wonderful way to stretch and massage the muscles and tendons on the bottom of your foot. This is a great therapeutic exercise for plantar fascia and other issues causing foot pain. The use of different size balls will change the intensity of pressure on your foot. Move slowly onto the ball, making sure to not to place your entire body weight on top.

MUSCLES BETWEEN YOUR TOES

- Place smooth rocks or spacers in between your toes.
- I particularly like doing this with the rocks warmed. You can accomplish this by placing the rocks in hot water. Just ensure that the rocks are not too hot.

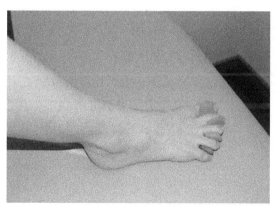

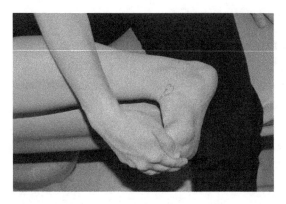

BOTTOM OF FOOT

- Sitting in an upright position, place your ankle on your knee.
- Grasp underneath your toes and slowly pull your toes up.

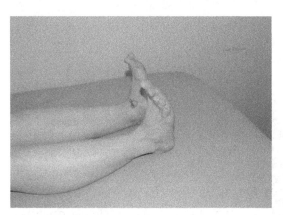

ANKLE, FEET, AND CALF

- You can perform this simple dynamic stretch sitting on the floor or in a chair.
- With your legs straight out in front of you, point your toes as far as you can, hold for a second or two, and then pull your toes toward you as far as you can. Repeat this 10-15 times.

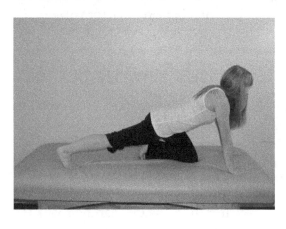

CALF AND BOTTOM OF THE FOOT

- Start this stretch from your hands and knees.
- Take one leg straight back and place toes on the floor.
- Slowly lean back into your back foot.
- Though you may feel this in your calf as well, ensure that you are focusing on stretching the bottom of the foot.

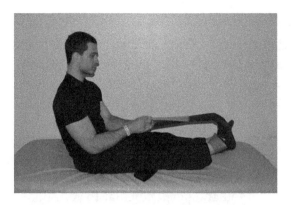

- In a seated position, place the TStretch strap around your ankle and up the bottom of your foot.
- Keeping your posture nice and tall, relax your foot and pull the strap toward you.

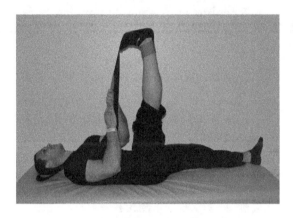

- Lying flat on your back, place the TStretch strap around your ankle and up the bottom of your foot.
- Bring your leg straight up and pull back and down on the strap.

HAMSTRING

- Lying on your back, place the TStretch strap around your ankle and up the bottom of your foot.
- Keeping your leg straight, pull your leg towards you.

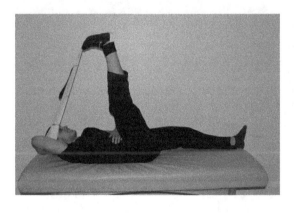

NECK AND SHOULDER STIFFNESS STRETCHING ROUTINE

Many times, when we are dealing with the stiffness in the neck, our shoulders are part of the problem. Your shoulders and upper back should also be worked in order to effectively have a positive impact on your neck. This program was designed to help work on those difficult areas that can often times lead to headaches and dizziness.

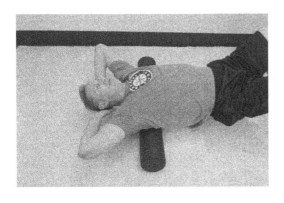

UPPER BACK

- Sit on the floor with the roller behind you and perpendicular to your body.
- Keeping your knees bent, lay back, placing the roller just above the midline.
- Raise your pelvis off the floor and slowly roll up and down your spine, ensuring that you do not take the roller lower than the rib cage.
- Relax your body and take the shape of the roller.

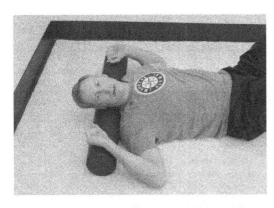

NECK

- Rolling your neck is very simple and feels great. Lying flat on your back, place the roller underneath your neck. The roller will be as close to your shoulders as possible.
- Roll your head to the right and then to the left. Pausing at any tender areas along the way.

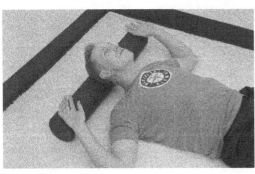

- Place the roller on the back of your head, just above the area where your neck and head attach. You may have to play with placement to get this just right.
- Start by pulling the roller in toward your body with your head. Your chin should be going straight up when you do this. Hold for 3-5 seconds.

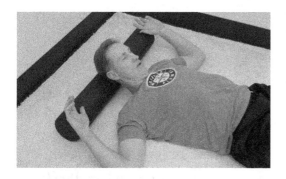

- Push the roller back out with your head. Your chin should be lowering down into your chest, stretching the back of your neck and into your upper back. Hold again and then repeat.

CHEST

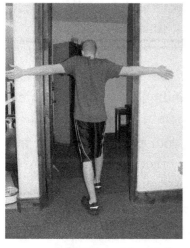

- Start by standing in a doorway. Straighten your arms and place them on each side of the doorway, approximately at shoulder height. Moving your hands up or down the doorway will change the angle of the stretch, so don't be afraid to experiment with your arm angle to feel what works best for you.
- Place one leg forward through the doorway.
- Keeping your posture nice and tall, slowly lean your body forward into the stretch.

UPPER BACK

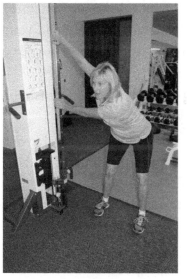

- Begin by standing with your side approximately one foot away from a door jamb or a secure post.
- With your feet shoulder width apart, grasp a door jamb or secure post with both hands (thumbs should point towards each other).
- Place the closest hand on the top about head height and the lower hand even with the lower portion of your chest.
- Making sure your hips are pointed forward, pull with your lower arm, and push with your upper arm.

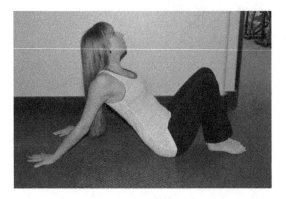

FRONT OF SHOULDERS AND BICEPS

- In a seated position, bend your knees and place your arms behind you.
- Slightly raise your rear end off the ground and slowly move toward your feet until you feel a stretch.
- Lower your rear end to the floor, keeping your back straight. Don't let your chest sink down.

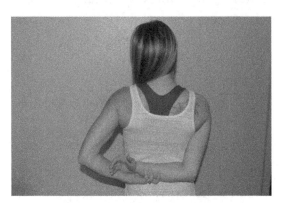

SHOULDER

- In a standing or seated position, place your arm behind your back.
- Keeping your posture nice and tall, use your other hand and pull your arm across your back.

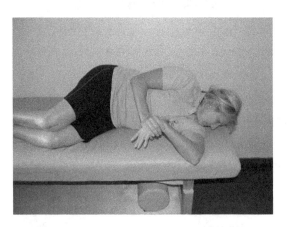

ROTATOR CUFF

- Lying on your side, bring your arm out to a 90-degree angle. Bend your elbow and wrist also to a 90-degree angle.
- Looking straight down, place your chin on your shoulder.
- Using your other hand, grab your wrist and gently push your elbow down into the ground. Slowly push your hand down toward the floor.

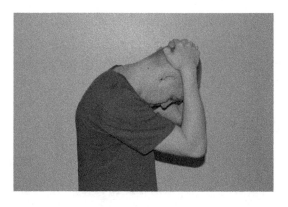

BACK OF NECK

- From a standing or seated position, interlock your hands behind your head.
- Keeping your posture nice and tall, slowly pull your head down.

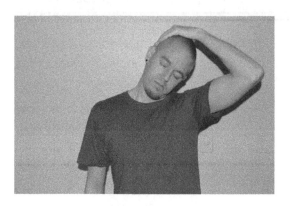

SIDE OF NECK

- In a standing or seated position, place your hand over the top of your head, grabbing the side of your head.
- Slowly pull your head to the side.

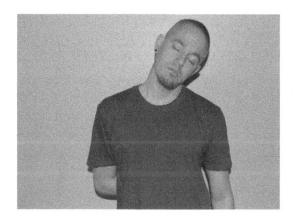

SIDE OF NECK AND SHOULDER

- In a standing or seated position, place your arm behind your back.
- Slowly lean your head to the other side until the stretch is felt.

NECK AND UPPER BACK STIFFNESS STRETCHING ROUTINE

By now, you are probably seeing a correlation between muscle groups and how one muscle group can affect another. This routine was designed to help those of you that may be dealing with neck and upper back pain. You will notice that I always try to start with the larger muscle groups first then we work on the smaller muscles. In this routine, we begin with the larger muscles of the upper back and then work on the neck.

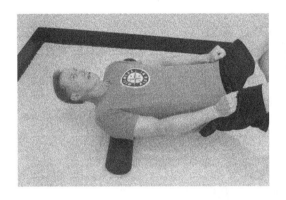

UPPER BACK

- Sit on the floor with the roller behind you and perpendicular to your body.
- Keeping your knees bent, lay back, placing the roller just above the midline.
- Raise your pelvis off the floor and slowly roll up and down your spine, ensuring that you do not take the roller lower than the rib cage.

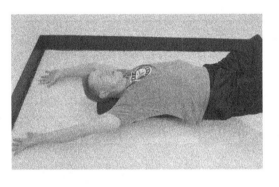

BACK

- Lie on the roller lengthwise with your head, upper back, and tailbone supported. Bend both knees and keep your feet flat on the floor for support.
- Draw your navel in and perform a pelvic tilt, laying your lower back on the roller.
- Just lying on the roller in this position with your hands on your chest may be enough.
- To add a little extra pressure to your upper back, bring your arms straight up above your head. Keep your lower back against the roller and relax.

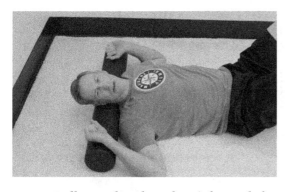

NECK

- Rolling your neck is very simple and feels great. Lying flat on your back, place the roller underneath your neck. The roller will be as close to your shoulders as possible.
- Close your eyes and just relax, taking deep breaths.
- Roll your head to the right and then to the left. Pausing at any tender areas along the way.

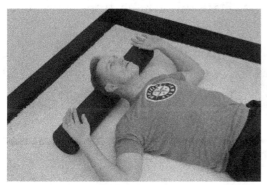 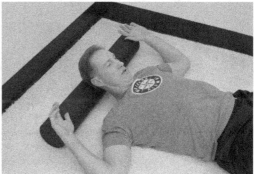

- Place the roller on the back of your head, just above the area where your neck and head attach. You may have to play with placement to get this just right.
- Start by pulling the roller in toward your body with your head. Your chin should be going straight up when you do this. Hold for 3-5 seconds.
- Push the roller back out with your head. Your chin should be lowering down into your chest, stretching the back of your neck and into your upper back. Hold again and then repeat.

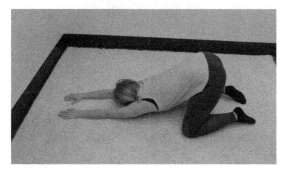

UPPER BACK

- On your hands and knees, slide your hands slightly in front of your head.
- Slowly move your chest down toward the ground, keeping your hips up.

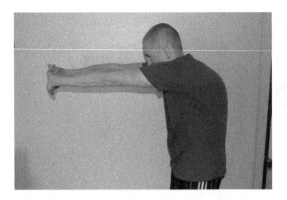

UPPER BACK

- In a standing or seated position, interlock your fingers.
- Extend your arms straight out in front of you with your palms facing out.
- Let your shoulders round forward.

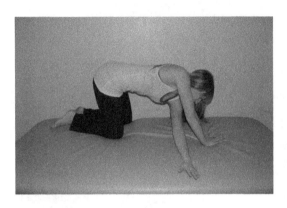

- Start this stretch from your hands and knees.
- Keeping one arm straight, slide your other arm under your body and lower your shoulder to the ground. Reach with the arm on the floor.
- Relax and hold the stretch, ensuring proper breathing.

- Begin by standing with your side approximately one foot away from a door jamb or a secure post.
- With your feet shoulder width apart, grasp a door jamb or secure post with both hands (thumbs should point towards each other).
- Place the closest hand on the top about head height and the lower hand even with the lower portion of your chest.
- Making sure your hips are pointed forward, pull with your lower arm, and push with your upper arm.

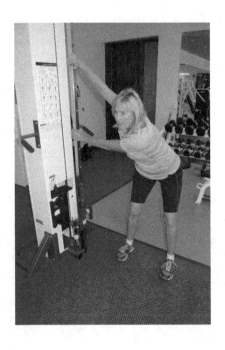

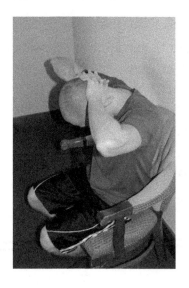

BACK OF NECK

- From a standing or seated position, interlock your hands behind your head.
- Keeping your posture nice and tall, slowly pull your head down.

SIDE OF NECK

- In a standing position, hold a weight or some sort of stationary object like a table. The idea is to keep your shoulder down.
- With the other hand, slowly pull the side of your head toward the floor.

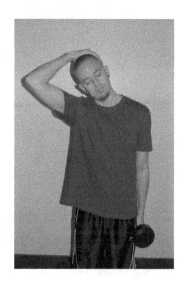

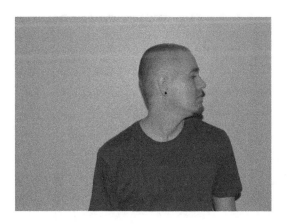

NECK

- In a standing or seated position, rotate your head to the side.
- Keep your posture nice and tall, and move your head slightly back to add a little more intensity.

HAND, WRIST, AND FOREARM STIFFNESS STRETCHING ROUTINE

We use our hands on a daily basis which causes tightness not just in our hands, but it can extend all the way up the wrist and into our forearm. This routine is a short routine that you can do virtually anywhere you are. I put this program together because we tend to forget this area of our body until it becomes a problem. You may find that these stretches are more difficult than you think, so move into them slowly.

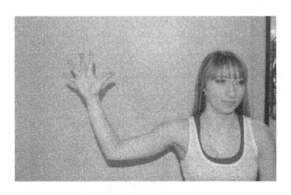

HAND AND FINGERS

- Open your hands and spread your fingers as far apart from each other as you can.

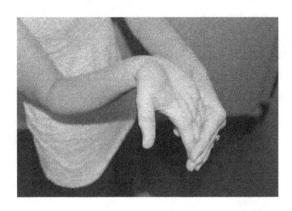

HAND AND WRIST

- Keeping your elbow bent and palm up, open your hand and keep your fingers together.
- Use your other hand to slowly pull back on your fingers.

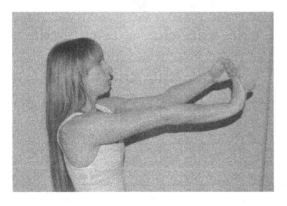

HAND, WRIST, FOREARM

- Keeping your arm straight out in front of you, open your hand and keep your fingers together and pointing upwards.
- Use your other hand to slowly pull back on your fingers.

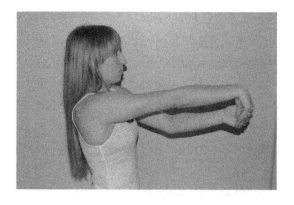

WRIST AND FOREARM

- Keeping your arm straight out in front of you, open your hand and keep your fingers together and pointing downwards.
- Use your other hand to slowly pull back on the back of your hand.

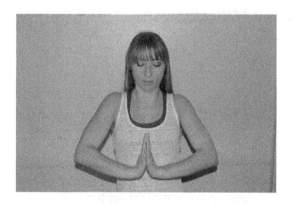

- Place the palms of your hands together.
- Slowly raise your elbows, keeping your palms together.

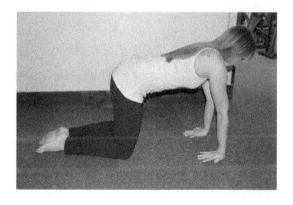

- Get on your hands and knees.
- Place your hands flat on the floor with your fingers pointed backward.
- Keeping the palms of your hands down on the floor, slowly move your body backward.

FOOT, ANKLE, AND SHIN STIFFNESS STRETCHING PROGRAM

Like our hands, our lower body and feet take a beating everyday. It is said that for every pound you weigh, you place five times that amount of weight on your feet and ankles; Wow! Like our hands, we tend to neglect this area of our body which can result in some major painful problems, such as plantar fasciitis, shin splints, and Achilles tendon problems. I am a big believer in working on an area before the problem begins. I hope everyone can take advantage of this program in some way.

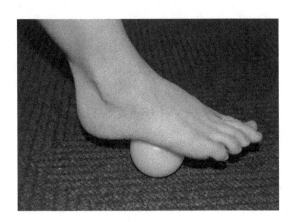

- Although this is not a foam roller, using a medium-size ball is a wonderful way to stretch and massage the muscles and tendons on the bottom of your foot. This is a great therapeutic exercise for plantar fascia and other issues causing foot pain. The use of different size balls will change the intensity of pressure on your foot. Move slowly onto the ball, making sure to not to place your entire body weight on top.

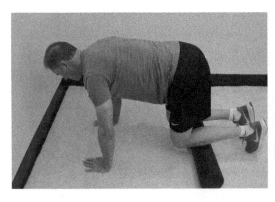
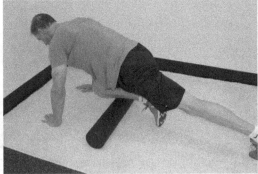

- A greatly overlooked area of the body is the shins. This is a wonderful exercise for people that like to run.
- The beginner starts by simply placing their hands on the floor while placing the foam roller approximately midway up the shin.
- Roll back and forth lengthwise up the shin to find those tender areas.

- The picture on the right shows a more advanced version, which puts more pressure on the muscle.
- Begin the second position by getting your hands set. Place one shin on the roller and rotate the foot so it points in and not down. Straighten out the other leg and place it behind you for stability and support.
- This position will also allow you to roll the lateral (outside) portion of the shin.

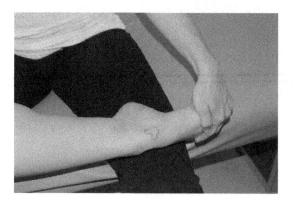

TOP OF FOOT, ANKLE, AND SHIN

- Sitting in an upright position, place your ankle on your knee.
- Grasp your toes at the top of the foot and slowly pull your toes down.

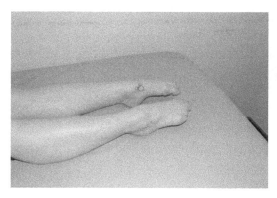
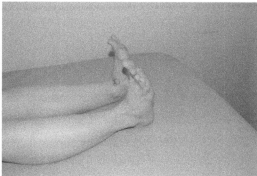

- You can perform this simple dynamic stretch sitting on the floor or in a chair.
- With your legs straight out in front of you, point your toes as far as you can, hold for a second or two, and then pull your toes toward you as far as you can. Repeat 10-15 times.

ANKLE

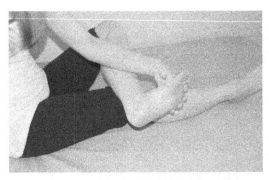
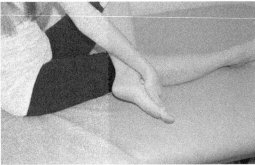

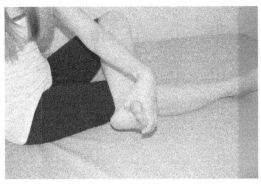

- Start off this stretch in a sitting position. Place an ankle on top of the opposite knee.
- Take hold of your foot and rotate your foot in a large circle.
- This stretch will take some time to learn how to do it properly. Many people want to help rotate the foot with the muscles that are supposed to be relaxed.
- Work on relaxing those muscles around your ankle while you manually rotate your foot. Repeat 10-15 times.

OUTSIDE OF ANKLE

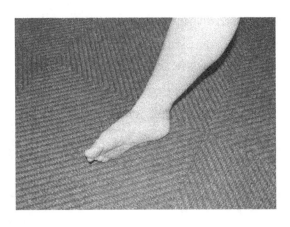

- Standing up with one leg slightly in front of the other, rotate on the outside of your foot.
- Slowly push down and feel the stretch on the outside of the foot and ankle.
- Hold the stretch, relax and ensure proper breathing. Hold on to a stable surface if you have balance issues. **Do not put all your weight down!**

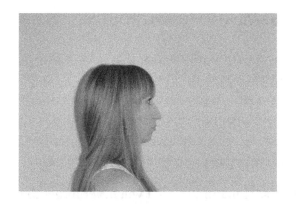

ANKLES AND SHINS

- Start this position on your knees with your toes pointed backward.
- Slowly sit down on your heels.

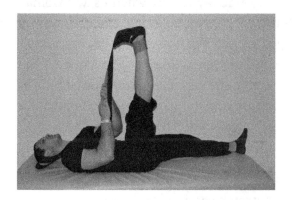

CALF AND ANKLE

- Lying flat on your back, place the TStretch strap around your ankle and up the bottom of your foot.
- Bring your leg straight up and pull back and down on the strap.

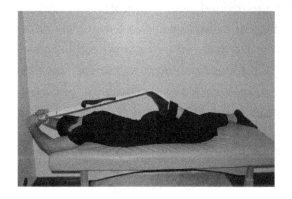

THIGH, TOP OF FOOT, SHIN

- Place a TStretch strap around your foot and lie flat on your stomach.
- Holding the strap with both hands, begin to pull your foot up toward your rear end.

PARKINSON'S DISEASE STATIC AND PASSIVE STRETCHING ROUTINE

I have had years of working with individuals with Parkinson's. If you have it, you understand how big of an affect it has on your body and how stiff you feel. I hope you also understand that moving your body is one of the best things you can do – it is crucial! This is why you are here now right? I designed this first program that is all static and passive stretches for you to just try to relax and focus on your breathing. Please take some time out of your schedule every day to do some sort of stretching.

Let me tell you a story about one of my clients, Muhammud Ali. I will never forget the night. I was pulling into the driveway of Harvey MacKay's house when I saw a woman sitting in the front seat of her car. She didn't see me pull in, as her attention was on something. I parked my car and as I was getting out, she was exiting her car as well. We simultaneously looked over at each other and she says, "You must be Aaron?" I was a little caught off guard because I didn't know who she was. She then followed it up by introducing herself, "I'm Lonnie Ali, I guess you are stretching me tonight". Again, I was caught off guard because I thought I was there to work with Harvey's wife, Carol Ann. I don't remember exactly what my words back to her were, but I was definitely EXCITED!

She made me feel comfortable from the minute we started talking as we walked into the house and throughout the entire 1 hour stretch session. As the session was finishing, Carol Ann came into the room and mentioned to us that dinner was ready. I honestly thought she was talking to Lonnie, but as I was walking toward the door, I noticed a place setting for me as well. We sat down and had a wonderful dinner, just talking about anything that came up. What I was oblivious to was the fact that Lonnie was actually interviewing me. She was making sure I was the right person to work with her husband, Muhammad. As our evening was coming to a close, Lonnie told me that Muhammad will love me, love the stretching and that, funny enough, he would also appreciate my size (6'2", 225 pounds). She also said that if he doesn't like it, he will just get off the table and walk away! What!?

It was a couple weeks later, and I was in Colorado Springs with my wife and her family when I got the call. It was Lonnie wanting to make an appointment for me to start working with Muhammad Ali. I didn't even have my appointment book with me at the time, but that didn't matter, I booked him. Now I couldn't wait to get back to Phoenix and start working with the champ. I did more researching on him than I had ever done before, learning more about his boxing career, his life after boxing, and of course his Parkinson's. I was actually very confident when I was heading over to his place. I had worked with professional athletes before and loved what I was doing, but I definitely didn't want him to get up off the table early and just walk away. Well, I ended up working with him for nearly 12 years, two times a week and I am happy to say he never left the table early...he did, however, run back to his chair when we were done.

Several years after I started working with him, I showed up on a Tuesday and there were photographers there. This wasn't necessarily abnormal, but what peaked my attention was that they were still there on Thursday when I showed up. The photographer approached me and said that he was amazed how much better Muhammad felt and walked after getting stretched on Tuesday. He asked me if he could take pictures of me stretching him for the magazine article. Absolutely, I said, not even knowing who he was or who he was working for. He ended up taking pictures for 45 minutes and the whole time, I was thinking, who is this man and why didn't I wear a shirt with my logo?

After the session was over, I walked into the kitchen with Muhammad as I hear the photographer and Lonnie talking about what issue the story was going to appear in. So I finally asked "What magazine are your photos for?" Lonnie immediately apologizes and introduces me to the photographer, Neil Leifer. She then goes on to tell me that Neil is the photographer that took the iconic photo of Muhammad standing over Sonny Liston. Wow! Neil extends his hand out to me and apologizes as well and tells me that the photos are going to be in Sports Illustrated. The issue was to celebrate Muhammad's 70th birthday and came out January 23, 2012, pg. 32 if you are interested. I can't even begin to explain how much I enjoyed working with and getting to know the Ali's! They are some of the most amazing and wonderful people I have ever met. I miss you Muhammad, thank you for everything!

This program is an all-around program that hits the entire body.

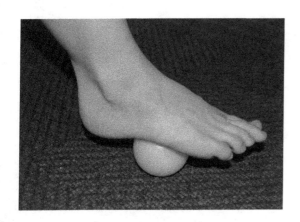

- Although this is not a foam roller, using a medium-size ball is a wonderful way to stretch and massage the muscles and tendons on the bottom of your foot. This is a great therapeutic exercise for plantar fascia and other issues causing foot pain. The use of different size balls will change the intensity of pressure on your foot. Move slowly onto the ball, making sure to not to place your entire body weight on top.

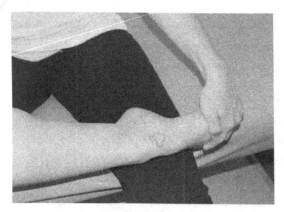

TOP OF FOOT, ANKLE, SHIN

- Sitting in an upright position, place your ankle on your knee.
- Grasp your toes at the top of the foot and slowly pull your toes down.

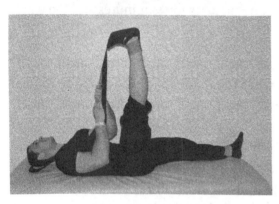

CALF AND ANKLE

- Lying flat on your back, place the TStretch strap around your ankle and up the bottom of your foot.
- Bring your leg straight up and pull back and down on the strap.

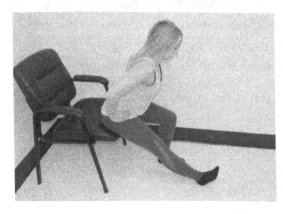

HAMSTRING

- Sit toward the end of a chair with one leg bent and the other leg straight out with the heel on the floor.
- Keeping your posture nice and tall, bend forward at the hips until you reach a stretched position. Do not hunch your back.

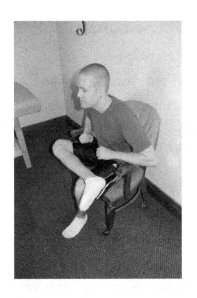

GLUTES AND LOWER BACK (SEATED POSITION)

- In a seated position, place your right ankle on your left knee.
- Keeping your posture nice and tall, slowly lean forward at the hips.

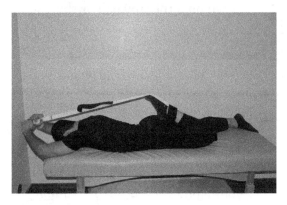

THIGH, SHIN, ANKLE

- Place a TStretch strap around your foot and lie flat on your stomach.
- Holding the strap with both hands, begin to pull your foot up toward your rear end.

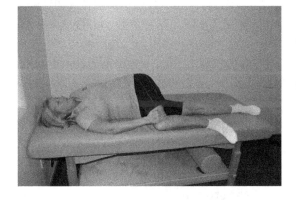

GLUTES AND LOWER BACK

- Lie on your side, bend your top leg and place it at a 90-degree angle.
- Slowly push your top shoulder back to the ground, holding your upper knee down to the floor.

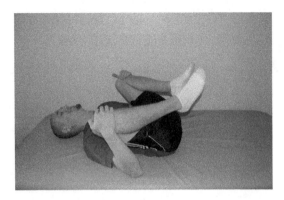

LOWER BACK

- Lie on your back.
- Pull both knees up toward your chest.
- Grasping your knees with your hands, pull your knees in toward your chest and out away from each other.

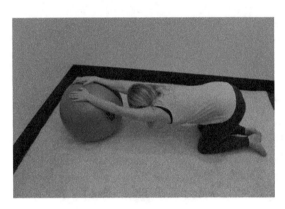

UPPER BACK

- While on your knees, place your arms straight out with your palms down on a therapy ball or the seat of a chair.
- Keeping your arms straight, slowly lower your chest to the ground.

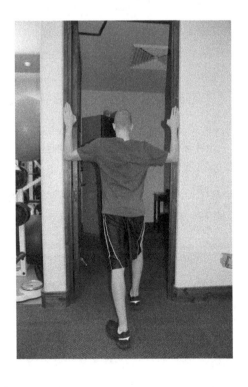

CHEST

- Start by standing in a doorway. Bend your elbows to a 90-degree angle.
- Place your hands and elbows on each side of the doorway. I try to keep my elbows up at shoulder height. Changing the height will change the angle of the stretch.
- Place one leg forward through the doorway.
- Keeping your posture nice and tall, slowly lean your body forward into the stretch.

BACK OF NECK

- From a standing or seated position, interlock your hands behind your head.
- Keeping your posture nice and tall, slowly pull your head down.

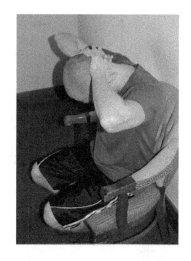

SIDE OF NECK

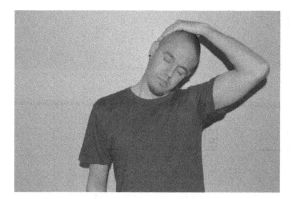

- In a standing or seated position, place your hand over the top of your head, grabbing the side of your head.
- Slowly pull your head to the side.

SIDE OF NECK AND SHOULDER

- In a standing or seated position, place your arm behind your back.
- Slowly lean your head to the other side until the stretch is felt.

PARKINSON'S DISEASE DYNAMIC STRETCHING ROUTINE

This routine focuses more on dynamic stretching and was made for you to get a little workout in as well as a great stretch. When doing this program I want you to really focus on getting as much out of each motion as you can. Focus on getting your foot higher, your rotation bigger, and your reach further with each repetition, while always focusing on being safe. If you would like to turn this in to a little workout, perform each dynamic stretch 2-3 times. I did add a few static stretches at the end for you to relax a little bit.

HIP FLEXOR, HAMSTRING, GLUTES

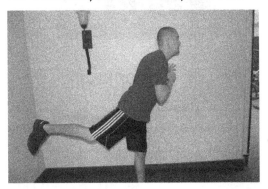

- Standing next to something stable for support and balance, swing your leg forward to get a stretch in your hamstring.
- Immediately swing your leg back behind you, stretching your hip flexors.

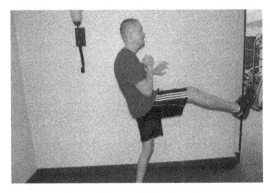

- Ensure proper breathing and repeat this stretch 10-15 times with each leg.
- Hold on to something stable for support and balance if needed.

ADDUCTORS AND HIPS

- Hold on to a stable object for support and balance.
- Standing approximately 2-3 feet away from support, bring one leg forward.
- Swing your leg across your body and out to the side, safely trying to get as much movement in your hip as possible. Repeat 10-15 times.

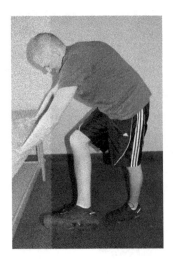

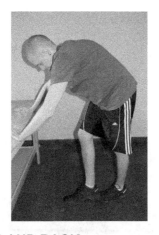 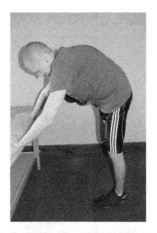

SHOULDERS AND BACK

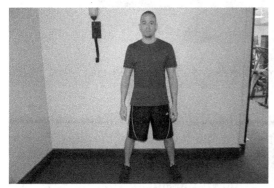 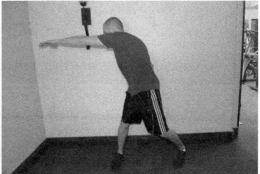

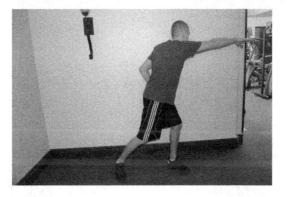

- Stand with your feet approximately shoulder-width apart.
- Turn your body and, with your left hand, reach as far as you can to your right side, then immediately turn back and reach with your right hand as far as you can to your left side.
- This stretch can be felt all the way down the side of your reaching arm and down into the lower back. Repeat 10-15 times each direction.

SHOULDERS, SIDE OF YOUR BODY, ADDUCTORS

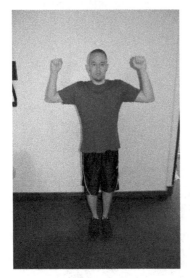 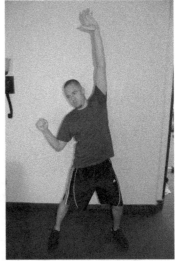

- Start with your feet together and both hands up with your elbows at shoulder height.
- Step out past shoulder-width with your left foot and raise your left arm high above your head. Return to the starting position and repeat on your right side, each time ensuring you are reaching as high into the sky as you possibly can. Don't get lazy.
- You should feel this stretch all the way down the side of your outstretched arm. Repeat 10-15 times.

BACK, CHEST, AND SHOULDERS

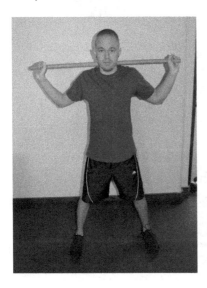 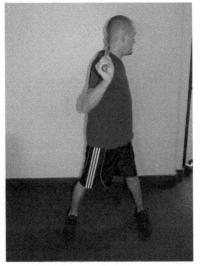

- Stand with your feet approximately shoulder-width apart.
- Carefully place and hold a pole of some sort on your upper back and shoulders.
- Keeping your posture nice and tall, rotate your upper body to the side. Repeat 10-15 times each direction.

LOWER BACK, HIPS, HAMSTRINGS

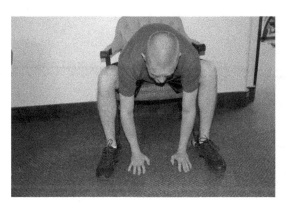

- Sit in a chair with your feet and knees wider than shoulder width.
- Keeping your posture nice and tall, slowly lower to the floor in between your knees and feet.
- To turn this into an exercise, raise back up with your hands in the air, then repeat lowering to the floor. Repeat 10-15 times. Hold the stretch at the end.

CALF

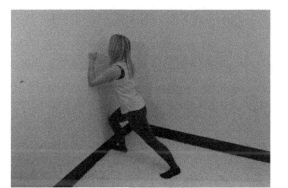

- Begin this stretch by placing the toes of one of your feet at the base of the wall.
- Placing both elbows on the wall, place your other foot a couple of feet behind you with toes pointed forward.
- Slowly lean a bit forward and down, taking your front knee and moving it toward the wall.
- Keep the heel of your back foot on the ground.
- If you can take your front knee to the wall without feeling a stretch, move your back foot back.

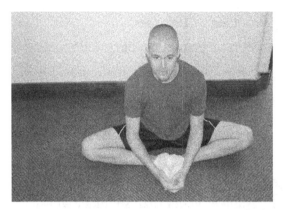

ADDUCTORS

- In a seated position, bend your knees and bring the bottom of your feet together.
- Sitting nice and tall, pull your feet in close to your body.
- Let your knees lay down to the ground.

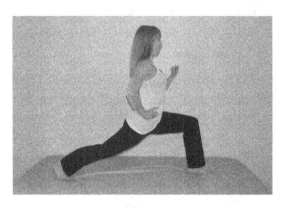

HIP FLEXOR AND HAMSTRING

- Standing with your feet together, place one leg forward into a lunge position.
- Keeping your back leg straight and your forward knee above your heel, move your weight down toward the ground. Ensure your posture is nice and tall.

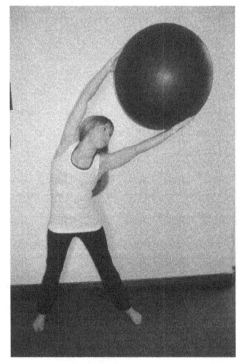

UPPER BACK AND SIDE OF YOUR BODY

- Stand with your feet approximately shoulder-width apart.
- Holding on to a therapy ball, extend your arms over your head.
- Keeping your posture nice and tall, lean to the side and focus on pushing the ball up and away from your body.

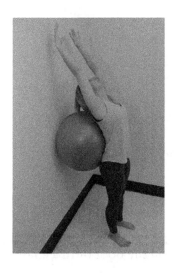

ABDOMINALS AND LOWER BACK

- Place a therapy ball against the wall.
- Position the ball so that you are resting your lower to mid back against the ball.
- With your hands stretched up above your head or hands behind your head, lean back against the ball. I tell my clients to try to take the shape of the ball and get your head up. Look up at the ceiling.

SEATED POSITION STRETCHING ROUTINE

I put this program together for the person that would still like to stretch but has a difficult time standing. This entire program is done while sitting in a chair. We are able to target most of the muscles in the body, however, the muscles in the front like your abdominals, hip flexors, and thighs are difficult to reach. We will be able to target your feet, calves, hamstrings, lower back, shoulders, and neck.

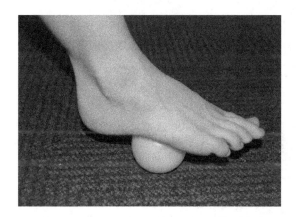

- Although this is not a foam roller, using a medium-size ball is a wonderful way to stretch and massage the muscles and tendons on the bottom of your foot. This is a great therapeutic exercise for plantar fascia and other issues causing foot pain. The use of different size balls will change the intensity of pressure on your foot. Move slowly onto the ball, making sure to not to place your entire body weight on top.

SHINS AND ANKLES

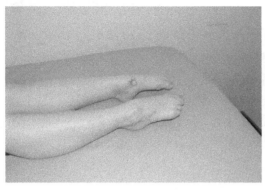 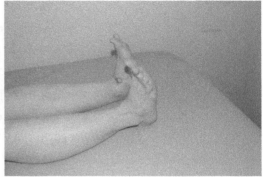

- You can perform this simple dynamic stretch sitting on the floor or in a chair.
- With your legs straight out in front of you, point your toes as far as you can, hold for a second or two, and then pull your toes toward you as far as you can. Repeat 10-15 times.

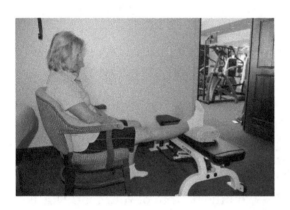

CALF AND HAMSTRING

- Sit in a chair with another chair or stationary object in front of you. Place a rolled-up towel on the chair in front of you.
- Put your foot on top of the towel and relax your knee down toward the ground.

CALF

- In a seated position, place the TStretch strap around your ankle and up the bottom of your foot.
- Keeping your posture nice and tall, relax your foot and pull the strap toward you.

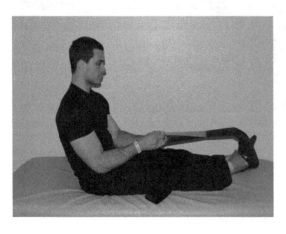

GLUTES AND LOWER BACK

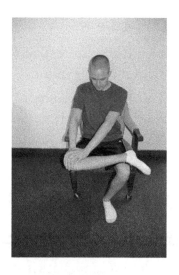

- In a seated position, place your right ankle on your left knee.
- Sitting in a nice and tall position, slowly push your right knee.

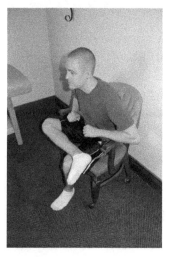

- While still seated, keep your right ankle over your left knee.
- Sitting nice and tall, slowly lean forward over your leg until you feel the stretch.

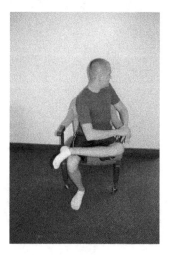

- In a seated position, place your left ankle on your right knee.
- Keeping your posture tall, slowly rotate your upper body to the left.

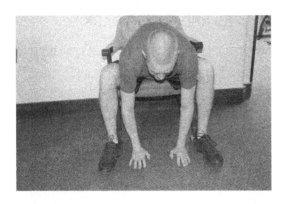

LOWER BACK

- Sit in a chair with your feet and knees wider than shoulder width.
- Keeping your posture nice and tall, slowly lower to the floor in between your knees and feet.

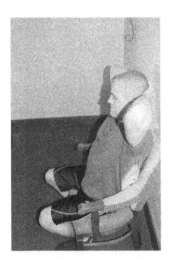

MID – BACK, ABDOMINALS, AND CHEST

- Sitting in a chair, roll up a bath towel and place it at your mid back.
- Place your hands on the back of your head.
- Keeping your posture nice and tall, slowly arch back into the towel.

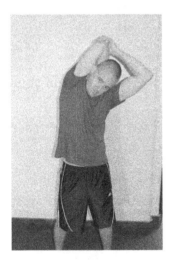

TRICEP AND UPPER BACK

- Keep your posture nice and tall from either a standing or sitting position.
- Pull your elbow over your head.
- Grab your elbow and pull back. Slowly lean your upper body to the side.

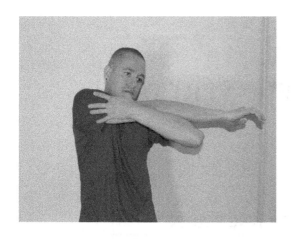

BACK OF SHOULDER AND UPPER BACK

- Keep your posture nice and tall from either a standing or sitting position.
- Reach across your body with your arm.
- With the other hand, grab the back of your arm.
- Pull your arm slightly out toward the other side of your body.

BACK OF NECK AND UPPER BACK

- Keep your posture nice and tall from either a standing or sitting position.
- Interlock your fingers and place them on the back of your head.
- Slowly pull your head down.
- Relax and hold the stretch, ensuring proper breathing.
- If you slowly move your elbows forward and slightly round your shoulders, you will feel the stretch moving down from your neck into your upper back.

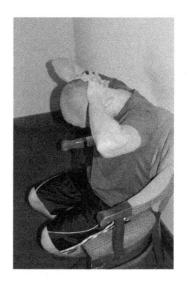

SIDE OF THE NECK

- In a standing or seated position, place your hand over the top of your head, grabbing the side of your head.
- Slowly pull your head to the side.

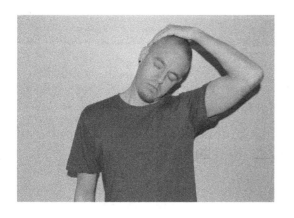

SPORTS SPECIFIC STRETCHES

BASEBALL PASSIVE AND STATIC STRETCHING ROUTINE

CALF

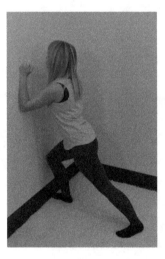

- Begin this stretch by placing the toes of one of your feet at the base of the wall.
- Placing both elbows on the wall, place your other foot a couple of feet behind you with toes pointed forward.
- Slowly lean a bit forward and down, taking your front knee and moving it toward the wall.
- Keep the heel of your back foot on the ground.
- If you can take your front knee to the wall without feeling a stretch, move your back foot back.

HAMSTRINGS

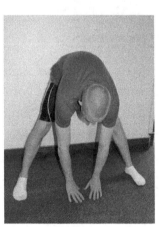

- Stand with your legs straight and feet a little wider than shoulder-width apart.
- Keeping a nice tall posture, bend forward at the hips.
- If you are unable to touch the floor, grasp behind your legs and hold.
- If you are able to touch the floor, work on placing your palms on the floor (don't force it).

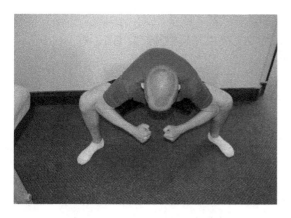

ADDUCTORS

- Stand with your feet approximately three feet apart.
- Squat down, keeping your knees above your heels.
- Place your elbows on the inside of your knees and push out.

THIGH

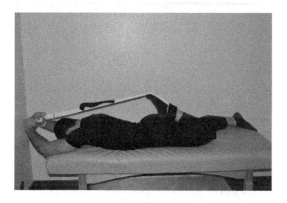

- Place a TStretch strap around your foot and lie flat on your stomach.
- Holding the strap with both hands, begin to pull your foot up toward your rear end.

HIP FLEXOR

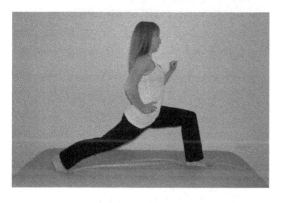

- Standing with your feet together, place one leg forward into a lunge position.
- Keeping your back leg straight and your forward knee above your heel, move your weight down toward the ground. Ensure your posture is nice and tall.

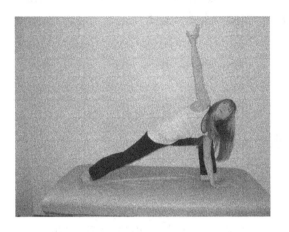

HIP FLEXOR, HAMSTRING, LOWER BACK

- Place your left leg forward into a lunge position.
- Keeping your right leg straight and your left knee above your heel, lean forward at the hips and place your left hand on the inside of your left foot.
- Pushing your left elbow into your knee, turn your body, and reach to the sky with your right arm.

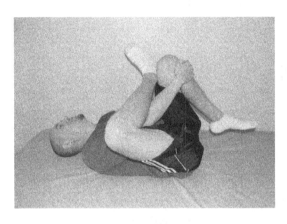

GLUTES

- Lie on your back with both knees bent.
- Place your right ankle on your left knee.
- Take your right arm through your legs and grasp your knee. Take your left hand and place it on your right hand, interlocking your fingers.
- Pull your left knee toward your chest, feeling this stretch in your right hip.

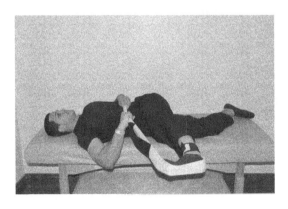

GLUTES AND LOWER BACK

- Place a TStretch strap around your left foot and lie on your right side.
- Holding the strap, keep your left leg straight.
- Slowly push your left shoulder back on the floor/ bed and pull your left leg up toward your head.

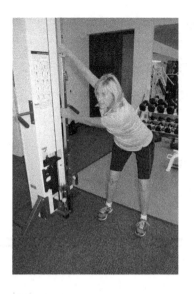

UPPER BACK

- Begin by standing with your side approximately one foot away from a door jamb or a secure post.
- With your feet shoulder width apart, grasp a door jamb or secure post with both hands (thumbs should point towards each other).
- Place the closest hand on the top about head height and the lower hand even with the lower portion of your chest.
- Making sure your hips are pointed forward, pull with your lower arm, and push with your upper arm.

ROTATOR CUFF

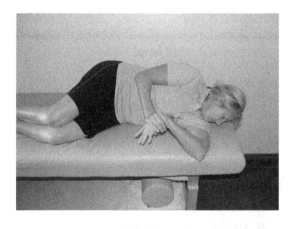

- Lying on your side, bring your arm out to a 90-degree angle. Bend your elbow and wrist also to a 90-degree angle.
- Looking straight down, place your chin on your shoulder.
- Using your other hand, grab your wrist and gently push your elbow down into the ground. Slowly push your hand down toward the floor.

FOREARMS AND WRISTS

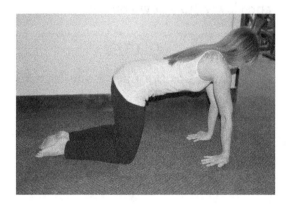

- Get on your hands and knees.
- Place your hands flat on the floor with your fingers pointed backward.
- Keeping the palms of your hands down on the floor, slowly move your body backward.

BASKETBALL PASSIVE AND STATIC STRETCHING ROUTINE

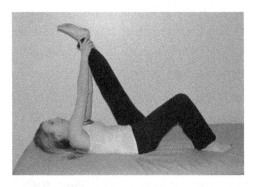

LOWER HAMSTRING

- Lie on your back, bend one knee so the bottom of your foot rests flat on the floor.
- Raise the other leg off the floor and grasp the lower portion of your calf.
- Keep your leg straight while pulling it towards you.

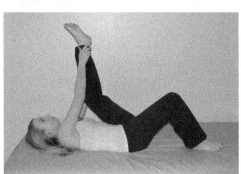

UPPER HAMSTRING

- Lie on your back with the bottom of one foot flat on the floor or bed.
- Raise your other leg off the floor and grasp the lower portion of your calf.
- With your knee bent, pull your leg down and toward your head.

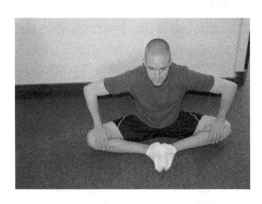

ADDUCTORS

- In a seated position, bend your knees and bring the bottom of your feet together.
- Sitting nice and tall, pull your feet in close to your body.
- Let your knees relax down to the ground and slowly push down on your knees.

GLUTES

- In a seated position, bend one leg and place it behind you and bend your forward leg to a 90-degree angle.
- Keeping your posture nice and tall, lean forward toward your knee.

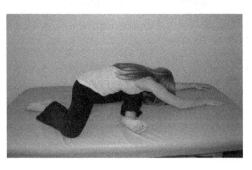

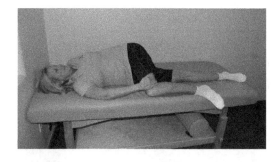

GLUTES AND LOWER BACK

- Lie on your side, bend your top leg and place it at a 90-degree angle.
- Slowly push your top shoulder back to the ground, holding your upper knee down to the floor.

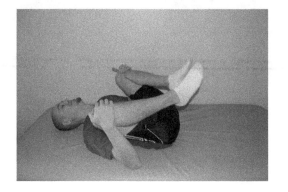

- Lie on your back.
- Pull both knees up toward your chest.
- Grasping your knees with your hands, pull your knees in toward your chest and out away from each other.

HIP FLEXOR, HAMSTRING, AND THIGH

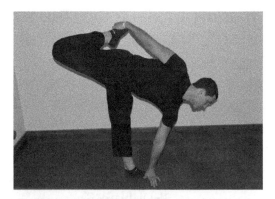

- In a standing position, grab a foot and pull it up to your rear end.
- Keeping hold of your foot, slowly lean forward and touch your hand to the floor.
- Keep your posture nice and tall.

UPPER BACK

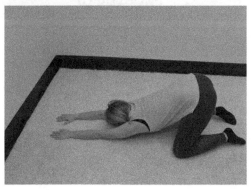

- On your hands and knees, slide your hands slightly in front of your head.
- Slowly move your chest down toward the ground keeping your hips up.

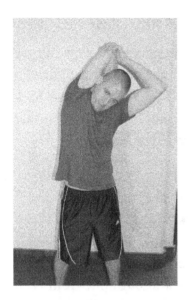

TRICEP AND UPPER BACK

- Keep your posture nice and tall from either a standing or sitting position.
- Pull your elbow over your head.
- Grab your elbow and pull back. Slowly lean your upper body to the side.

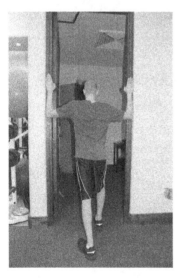

CHEST

- Start by standing in a doorway. Bend your elbows to a 90- degree angle.
- Place your hands and elbows on each side of the doorway. I try to keep my elbows up at shoulder height. Changing the height will change the angle of the stretch.
- Place one leg forward through the doorway.
- Keeping your posture nice and tall, slowly lean your body forward into the stretch.

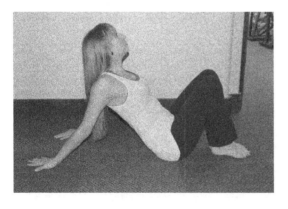

SHOULDERS

- In a seated position, bend your knees and place your arms behind you.
- Slightly raise your rear end off the ground and slowly move toward your feet until you feel a stretch.
- Lower your rear end to the floor, keeping your back straight. Don't let your chest sink down.

BOWLING PASSIVE AND STATIC STRETCHING ROUTINE

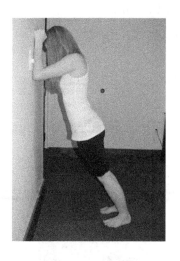

CALVES

- Standing approximately an arm's length away from the wall, stand with your feet about six inches apart with toes pointed forward.
- Lean on the wall with both elbows. Ensure that you keep a straight line with your knees, hips, back, and neck. Do not let your hips sink in toward the wall.
- Stand with both heels on the ground.
- If your heels are on the ground and you do not feel a stretch, move back.

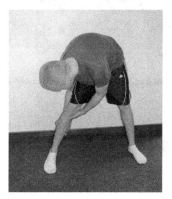

HAMSTRING

- Stand with your legs straight and a little wider than shoulder-width apart.
- Keeping your posture nice and tall, bend forward at the hips toward the right side.
- Grasp behind the leg and pull down slightly.

HIP FLEXOR, GLUTES, LOWER BACK

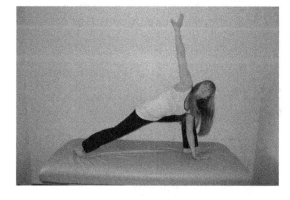

- Place your left leg forward into a lunge position.
- Keeping your right leg straight and your left knee above your heel, lean forward at the hips and place your left hand on the inside of your left foot.
- Pushing your left elbow into your knee, turn your body, and reach to the sky with your right arm.

GLUTES

- From a seated position, bend your knee with your foot behind you.
- Bend your opposite leg in front of you and place your foot against the other knee.
- Keeping your posture tall, bend forward at your hips.
- Relax and hold the stretch, ensuring proper breathing.
- This is a great stretch because you can lean forward in different directions and stretch different muscles in the hip.

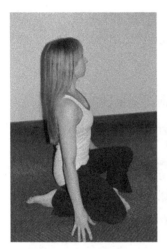 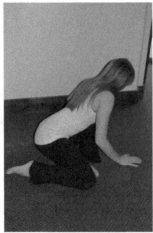 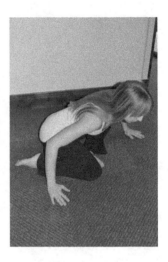

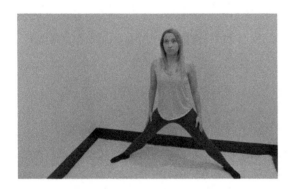

ADDUCTORS

- In a standing position, slowly spread your feet apart until you feel the stretch in between your legs.
- Keep your posture nice and tall.
- Relax and hold the position, ensuring proper breathing.

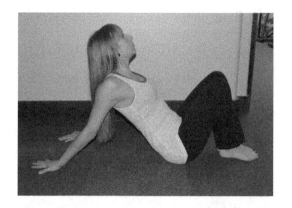

SHOULDERS AND BICEPS

- In a seated position, bend your knees and place your arms behind you.
- Slightly raise your rear end off the ground and slowly move toward your feet until you feel a stretch.
- Lower your rear end to the floor, keeping your back straight. Don't let your chest sink down.

HAND, WRIST, AND FOREARM

- Keeping your arm straight out in front of you, open your hand and keep your fingers together and pointing upwards.
- Use your other hand to slowly pull back on your fingers.

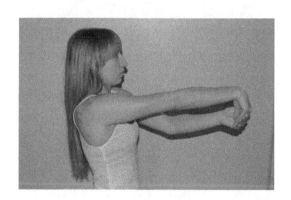

WRIST AND FOREARM

- Keeping your arm straight out in front of you, open your hand and keep your fingers together and pointing downwards.
- Use your other hand to slowly pull back on the back of your hand.

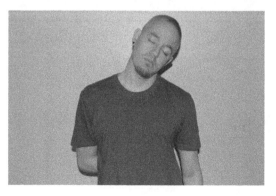

SHOULDER AND NECK

- In a standing or seated position, place your arm behind your back.
- Slowly lean your head to the other side until   the stretch is felt.

BOXING PASSIVE AND STATIC STRETCHING ROUTINE

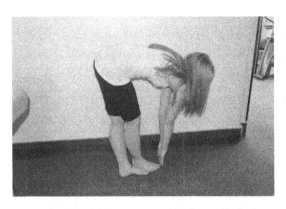

HAMSTRING AND CALF

- In a standing position, cross one leg in front of the other.
- Keeping your posture nice and tall (try not to arch the back), bend forward at the hips. This move will give you an intense stretch behind the knee.
- Relax and hold the stretch, ensuring proper breathing. Slowly rise up when you are done.

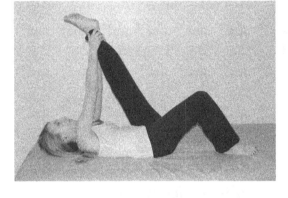

LOWER HAMSTRING

- Lie on your back, bend one knee so the bottom of your foot rests flat on the floor.
- Raise the other leg off the floor and grasp the lower portion of your calf.
- Keep your leg straight while pulling it towards you.

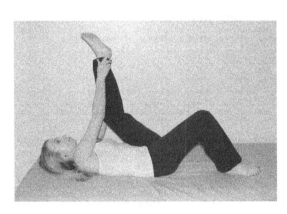

UPPER HAMSTRING

- Lie on your back with the bottom of one foot flat on the floor or bed.
- Raise your other leg off the floor and grasp the lower portion of your calf.
- With your knee bent, pull your leg down and toward your head.

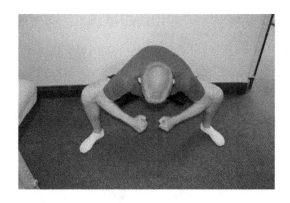

ADDUCTORS

- Stand with your feet approximately three feet apart.
- Squat down, keeping your knees above your heels.
- Place your elbows on the inside of your knees and push out.

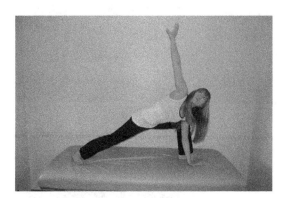

HIP FLEXOR, GLUTES, HAMSTRING, LOWER BACK

- Place your left leg forward into a lunge position.
- Keeping your right leg straight and your left knee above your heel, lean forward at the hips and place your left hand on the inside of your left foot.
- Pushing your left elbow into your knee, turn your body, and reach to the sky with your right arm.

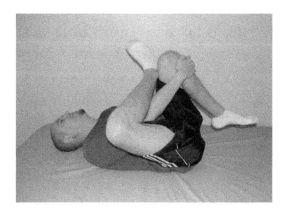

GLUTES

- Lie on your back with both knees bent.
- Place your right ankle on your left knee.
- Take your right arm through your legs and grasp your knee. Take your left hand and place it on your right hand, interlocking your fingers.
- Pull your left knee toward your chest, feeling this stretch in your right hip.

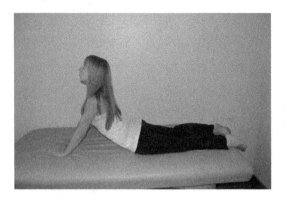

ABDOMINALS

- Lie on your stomach.
- Place your hands underneath your shoulders and rise up. Look straight ahead.
- Relax and hold the stretch, ensuring proper breathing.

UPPER BACK

- Begin by standing with your side approximately one foot away from a door jamb or a secure post.
- With your feet shoulder width apart, grasp a door jamb or secure post with both hands (thumbs should point towards each other).
- Place the closest hand on the top about head height and the lower hand even with the lower portion of your chest.
- Making sure your hips are pointed forward, pull with your lower arm, and push with your upper arm.

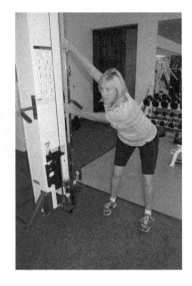

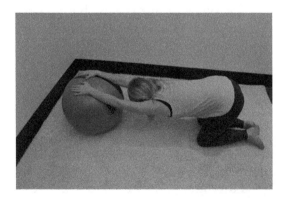

- While on your knees, place your arms straight out with your palms down on a therapy ball or chair.
- Keeping your arms straight, slowly lower your chest to the ground.

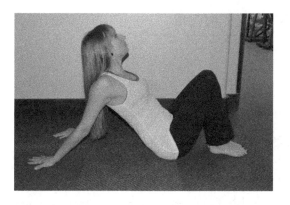

SHOULDERS AND BICEPS

- In a seated position, bend your knees and place your arms behind you.
- Slightly raise your rear end off the ground and slowly move toward your feet until you feel a stretch.
- Lower your rear end to the floor, keeping your back straight. Don't let your chest sink down.

BACK OF NECK AND UPPER BACK

- From a standing or seated position, interlock your hands behind your head.
- Keeping your posture nice and tall, slowly pull your head down.

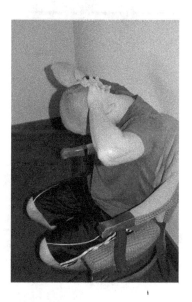

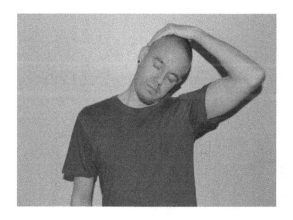

SIDE OF NECK

- In a standing or seated position, place your hand over the top of your head, grabbing the side of your head.
- Slowly pull your head to the side.

CYCLIST PASSIVE AND STATIC STRETCHING ROUTINE

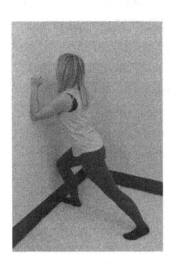

CALVES

- Begin this stretch by placing the toes of one of your feet at the base of the wall.
- Placing both elbows on the wall, place your other foot a couple of feet behind you with toes pointed forward.
- Slowly lean a bit forward and down, taking your front knee and moving it toward the wall.
- Keep the heel of your back foot on the ground.
- If you can take your front knee to the wall without feeling a stretch, move your back foot back.

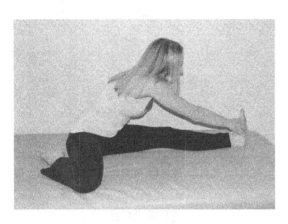

HAMSTRING

- In a seated position, place one leg straight out in front of you. Bend the other leg and place the foot behind you with your knee pointed out.
- Keeping your posture nice and tall, bend forward at the hips.
- Slowly reach for your toes.

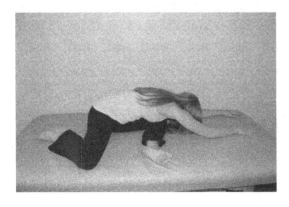

GLUTES

- In a seated position, bend one leg and place it behind you and bend your forward leg to a 90-degree angle.
- Keeping your posture nice and tall, lean forward toward your knee.

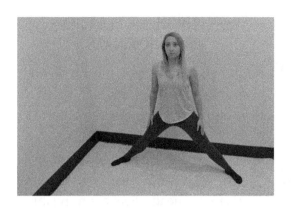

ADDUCTORS

- In a standing position, slowly spread your feet apart until you feel the stretch in between your legs.
- Keep your posture nice and tall.
- Relax and hold the position, ensuring proper breathing.

THIGH

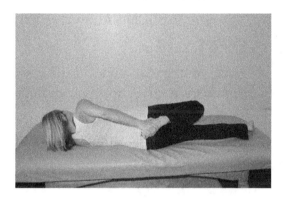

- Lie on your side.
- Bring one leg back and grab it with your hand.
- Pull your knee in toward your rear end, keeping it from moving forward.
- Keep your body from tipping forward.

THIGH AND HIP FLEXOR

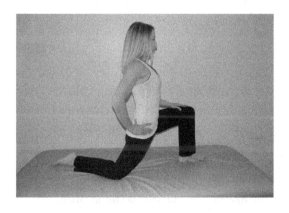

- Get down on both knees and place one foot forward in a lunge position.
- Take your weight down and forward, keeping your posture nice and tall.

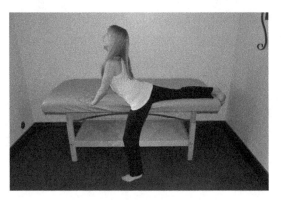

THIGH, HIP FLEXOR, ABDOMINALS

- Using your bed or table, lie on your stomach on the side of the table with one leg supporting you on the ground.
- Place your hands underneath your shoulders and rise up, looking straight ahead. Focus on pushing your thigh into the table.

ABDOMINALS

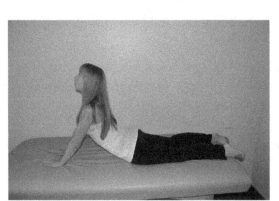

- Lie on your stomach.
- Place your hands underneath your shoulders and rise up. Look straight ahead.
- Relax and hold the stretch, ensuring proper breathing.
- This stretch can place a tremendous amount of stress on the lower back. If it is too much do this from your elbows.

UPPER BACK

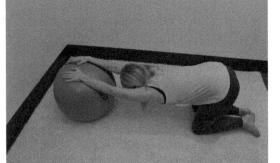

- While on your knees, place your arms straight out with your palms down on a therapy ball or seat of a chair.
- Keeping your arms straight, slowly lower your chest to the ground.

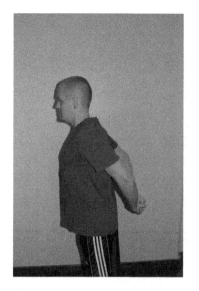

CHEST AND SHOULDERS

- In a standing position, take hold of your hands behind your back.
- Keeping your posture tall and looking forward, slowly push your hands back, away from your body. Think of pushing your chest out.

BACK OF NECK

- From a standing or seated position, interlock your hands behind your head.
- Keeping your posture nice and tall, slowly pull your head down.

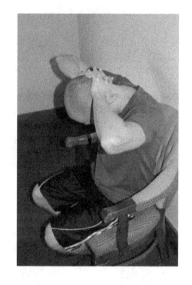

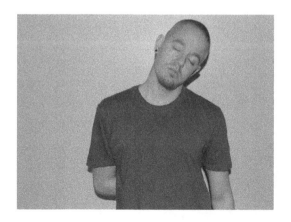

SHOULDER AND NECK

- In a standing or seated position, place your arm behind your back.
- Slowly lean your head to the other side until the stretch is felt.

FOOTBALL PASSIVE AND STATIC STRETCHING ROUTINE

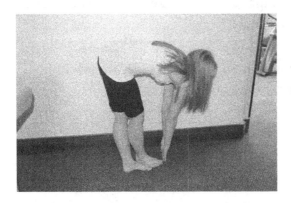

CALF AND HAMSTRING

- In a standing position, cross one leg in front of the other.
- Keeping your posture nice and tall (try not to arch the back), bend forward at the hips. This move will give you an intense stretch behind the knee.

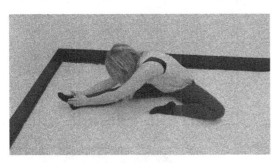

HAMSTRING

- In a seated position, straighten one leg and place it out into a splits position. Bend your other leg and bring your foot in close to your body.
- Keeping your posture nice and tall, bend toward the straightened leg.

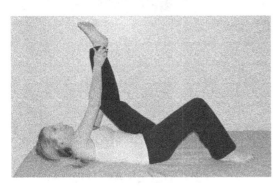

UPPER HAMSTRING

- Lie on your back with the bottom of one foot flat on the floor or bed.
- Raise your other leg off the floor and grasp the lower portion of your calf.
- With your knee bent, pull your leg down and toward your head.

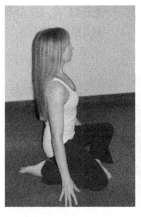 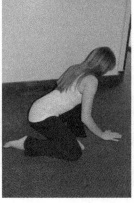 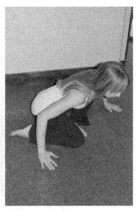

- From a seated position, bend your knee with your foot behind you.
- Bend your opposite leg in front of you and place your foot against the other knee.
- Keeping your posture tall, bend forward at your hips.
- This is a great stretch because you can lean forward in different directions and stretch different muscles in the hip.

ADDUCTORS

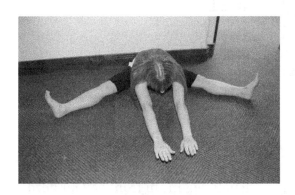

- In a seated position, spread your legs as far as they will go.
- Keeping your posture nice and tall and your toes pointed up, bend forward at the hips.

HIP FLEXOR, HAMSTRING, THIGH

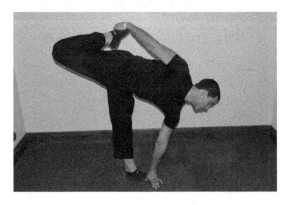

- In a standing position, grab a foot and pull it up to your rear end.
- Keeping hold of your foot, slowly lean forward and touch your hand to the floor.
- Keep your posture nice and tall.

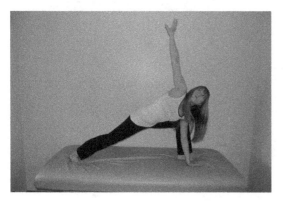

HIP FLEXOR, GLUTES, HAMSTRING

- Place your left leg forward into a lunge position.
- Keeping your right leg straight and your left knee above your heel, lean forward at the hips and place your left hand on the inside of your left foot.
- Pushing your left elbow into your knee, turn your body, and reach to the sky with your right arm.

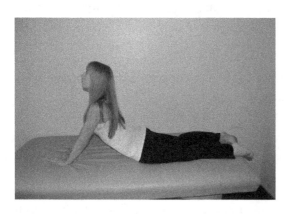

ABDOMINALS

- Lie on your stomach.
- Place your hands underneath your shoulders and rise up. Look straight ahead.
- Relax and hold the stretch, ensuring proper breathing.
- This stretch can place a tremendous amount of stress on the lower back.

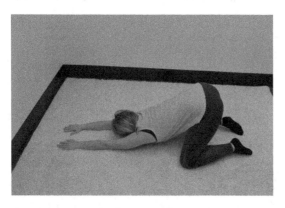

UPPER BACK

- On your hands and knees, slide your hands slightly in front of your head.
- Slowly move your chest down toward the ground keeping your hips up.

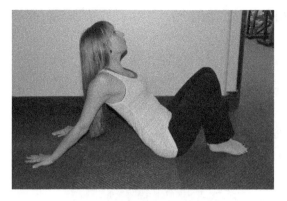

SHOULDERS AND BICEPS

- In a seated position, bend your knees and place your arms behind you.
- Slightly raise your rear end off the ground and slowly move toward your feet until you feel a stretch.
- Lower your rear end to the floor, keeping your back straight. Don't let your chest sink down.

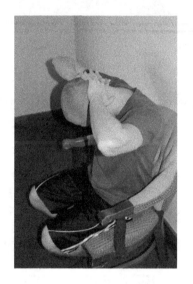

BACK OF NECK AND UPPER BACK

- From a standing or seated position, interlock your hands behind your head.
- Keeping your posture nice and tall, slowly pull your head down.
- Relax and hold the stretch, ensuring proper breathing.

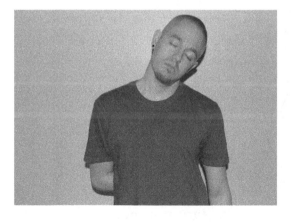

SHOULDER AND SIDE OF NECK

- In a standing or seated position, place your arm behind your back.
- Slowly lean your head to the other side until the stretch is felt.

GOLF PASSIVE AND STATIC STRETCHING ROUTINE

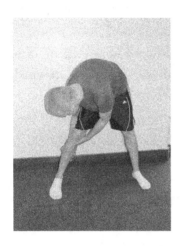

HAMSTRING

- Stand with your legs straight and a little wider than shoulder-width apart.
- Keeping your posture nice and tall, bend forward at the hips toward the right side.
- Grasp behind the leg and pull down slightly.

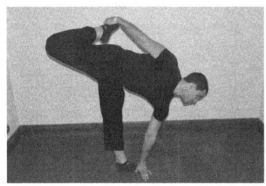

HAMSTRING, HIP FLEXOR, THIGH

- In a standing position, grab a foot and pull it up to your rear end.
- Keeping hold of your foot, slowly lean forward and touch your hand to the floor.
- Keep your posture nice and tall.

HIP FLEXOR, GLUTES, HAMSTRING

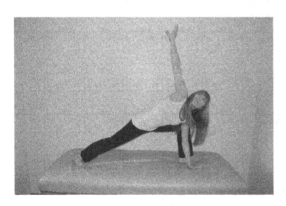

- Place your left leg forward into a lunge position.
- Keeping your right leg straight and your left knee above your heel, lean forward at the hips and place your left hand on the inside of your left foot.
- Pushing your left elbow into your knee, turn your body, and reach to the sky with your right arm.

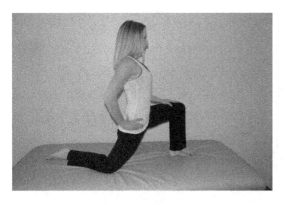

HIP FLEXOR AND THIGH

- Get down on both knees and place one foot forward in a lunge position.
- Take your weight down and forward, keeping your posture nice and tall.

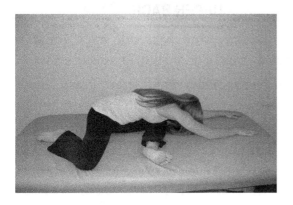

GLUTES

- In a seated position, bend one leg and place it behind you and bend your forward leg to a 90-degree angle.
- Keeping your posture nice and tall, lean forward toward your knee.

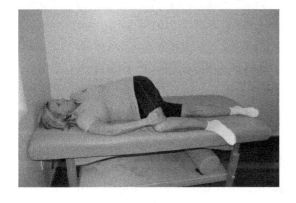

GLUTES AND LOWER BACK

- Lie on your side, bend your top leg and place it at a 90-degree angle.
- Slowly push your top shoulder back to the ground, holding your upper knee down to the floor.

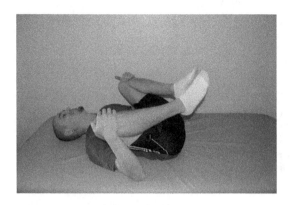

- Lie on your back.
- Pull both knees up toward your chest.
- Grasping your knees with your hands, pull your knees in toward your chest and out away from each other.

UPPER BACK

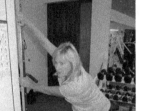

- Begin by standing with your side approximately one foot away from a door jamb or a secure post.
- With your feet shoulder width apart, grasp a door jamb or secure post with both hands (thumbs should point towards each other).
- Place the closest hand on the top about head height and the lower hand even with the lower portion of your chest.
- Making sure your hips are pointed forward, pull with your lower arm, and push with your upper arm. This is a great stretch for rotation!

BACK AND SIDE OF BODY

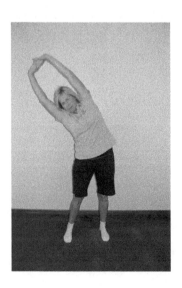

- Stand with your feet approximately shoulder-width apart.
- Interlock your fingers and raise your arms over your head.
- Keeping your posture nice and tall, lean to the side and focus on pushing the palms of your hands up and out away from your body.

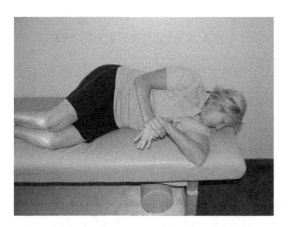

ROTATOR CUFF

- Lying on your side, bring your arm out to a 90-degree angle. Bend your elbow and wrist also to a 90-degree angle.

- Looking straight down, place your chin on your shoulder.

- Using your other hand, grab your wrist and gently push your elbow down into the ground. Slowly push your hand down toward the floor.

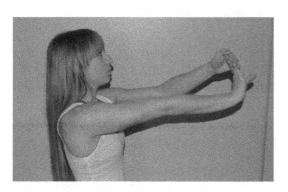

HAND, WRIST, AND FOREARM

- Keeping your arm straight out in front of you, open your hand and keep your fingers together and pointing upwards.

- Use your other hand to slowly pull back on your fingers.

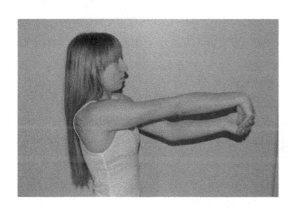

FOREARM AND WRIST

- Keeping your arm straight out in front of you, open your hand and keep your fingers together and pointing downwards.

- Use your other hand to slowly pull back on the back of your hand.

HOCKEY PASSIVE AND STATIC STRETCHING ROUTINE

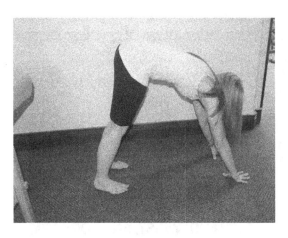

CALVES AND HAMSTRINGS

- Begin this stretch in a push up position.
- Slowly move your hands back toward your feet and lift your hips higher in the air.
- Slowly push your heels back into the ground.
- Relax and hold the stretch, ensuring proper breathing.

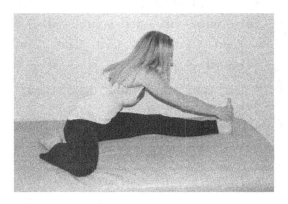

HAMSTRING

- In a seated position, place one leg straight out in front of you. Bend the other leg and place the foot behind you with your knee pointed out.
- Keeping your posture nice and tall, bend forward at the hips.
- Slowly reach for your toes.

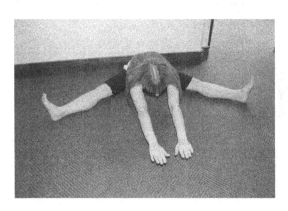

ADDUCTORS AND HAMSTRINGS

- In a seated position, spread your legs as far as they will go.
- Keeping your posture nice and tall and your toes pointed up, bend forward at the hips.

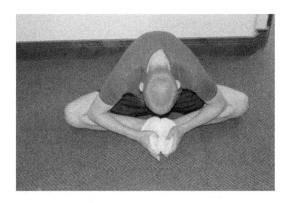

ADDUCTORS AND LOWER BACK

- In a seated position, bend your knees and bring the bottom of your feet together.
- Pull your feet in close to your body.
- Let your knees lay down to the ground. Pushing your knees down with your elbows, slowly lean forward.

GLUTES

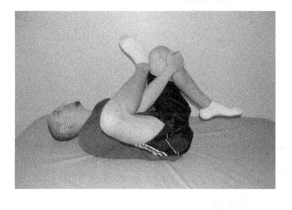

- Lie on your back with both knees bent.
- Place your right ankle on your left knee.
- Take your right arm through your legs and grasp your knee. Take your left hand and place it on your right hand, interlocking your fingers.
- Pull your left knee toward your chest, feeling this stretch in your right hip.

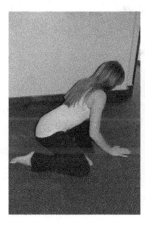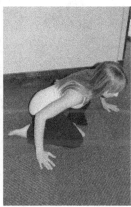

- From a seated position, bend your knee with your foot behind you.
- Bend your opposite leg in front of you and place your foot against the other knee.

- Keeping your posture tall, bend forward at your hips.
- Relax and hold the stretch, ensuring proper breathing. This is a great stretch because you can lean forward in different directions and stretch different muscles in the hip.

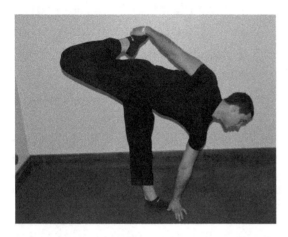

HAMSTRING, HIP FLEXOR, THIGH

- In a standing position, grab a foot and pull it up to your rear end.
- Keeping hold of your foot, slowly lean forward and touch your hand to the floor.
- Keep your posture nice and tall.

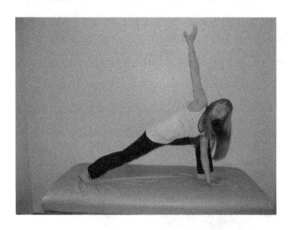

HIP FLEXOR, GLUTES, LOWER BACK

- Place your left leg forward into a lunge position.
- Keeping your right leg straight and your left knee above your heel, lean forward at the hips and place your left hand on the inside of your left foot.
- Pushing your left elbow into your knee, turn your body, and reach to the sky with your right arm.

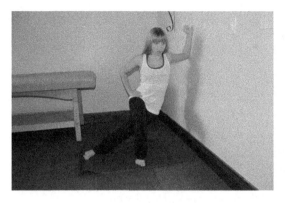

IT BAND AND HIP

- Stand approximately elbow length away from the wall.
- Take the leg closest to the wall and cross it behind you. Slide it away from the wall as you slowly lower down toward the ground. Do not let your forward knee get past your toes.

UPPER BACK, CHEST, ABDOMINALS

- Hold onto a bar overhead.
- Move your feet backward so your arms are reaching forward.
- Place your weight on your toes and lean forward into the stretch.

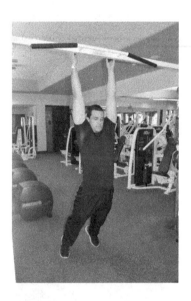

ABDOMINALS

- Lie on your stomach.
- Place your hands underneath your shoulders and rise up. Look straight ahead.
- Relax and hold the stretch, ensuring proper breathing.

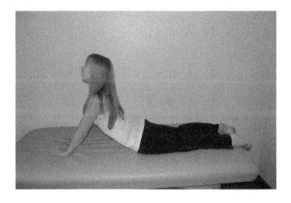

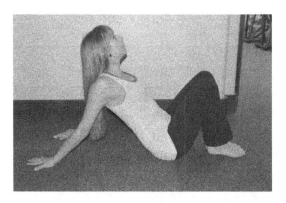

SHOULDERS AND BICEPS

- In a seated position, bend your knees and place your arms behind you.

- Slightly raise your rear end off the ground and slowly move toward your feet until you feel a stretch.

- Lower your rear end to the floor, keeping your back straight. Don't let your chest sink down.

UPPER BACK

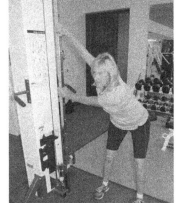

- Begin by standing with your side approximately one foot away from a door jamb or a secure post.

- With your feet shoulder width apart, grasp a door jamb or secure post with both hands (thumbs should point towards each other).

- Place the closest hand on the top about head height and the lower hand even with the lower portion of your chest.

- Making sure your hips are pointed forward, pull with your lower arm, and push with your upper arm.

RUNNERS PASSIVE AND STATIC STRETCHING ROUTINE

TOPS OF FEET AND SHINS

- Start this position on your knees with your toes pointed backward.
- Slowly sit down on your heels.

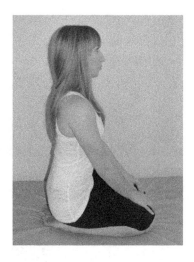

CALF

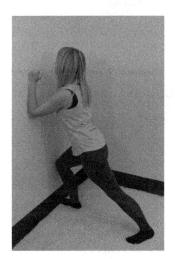

- Begin this stretch by placing the toes of one of your feet at the base of the wall.
- Placing both elbows on the wall, place your other foot a couple of feet behind you with toes pointed forward.
- Slowly lean a bit forward and down, taking your front knee and moving it toward the wall.
- Keep the heel of your back foot on the ground.
- If you can take your front knee to the wall without feeling a stretch, move your back foot back.

HAMSTRING

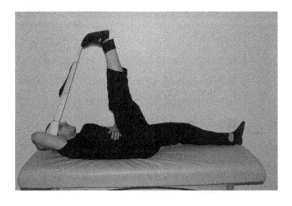

- Lying on your back, place the TStretch strap around your ankle and up the bottom of your foot.
- Keeping your leg straight, pull your leg towards you.

279

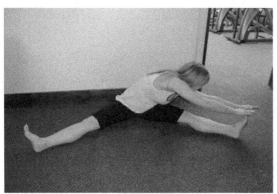

HAMSTRINGS AND ADDUCTORS

- In a seated position, spread your legs as far as they will let you go.
- Keeping your posture nice and tall and your toes pointed up, bend to one side.

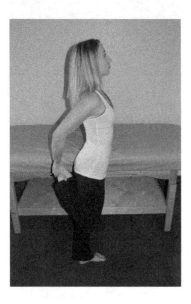

THIGH

- Stand with both feet together, keeping your posture nice and tall.
- Pick one leg up behind you, reach around and grab your foot.
- Pull your knee in toward your rear end. Try not to let your knee move forward.
- Keep your posture nice and tall, not letting your shoulder slump forward.

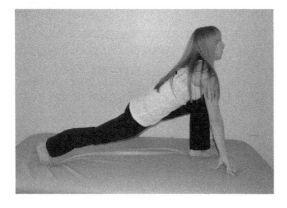

HIP FLEXOR, GLUTES, HAMSTRING

- Standing with your feet together, place one leg forward into a lunge position.
- Keeping your back leg straight and your forward knee above your heel, lean forward at the hips and place both hands on the ground.
- Move your weight down toward the ground.

GLUTES

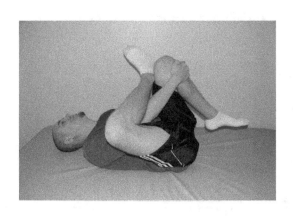

- Lie on your back with both knees bent.
- Place your right ankle on your left knee.
- Take your right arm through your legs and grasp your knee. Take your left hand and place it on your right hand, interlocking your fingers.
- Pull your left knee toward your chest, feeling this stretch in your right hip.

OUTSIDE OF HIP AND UPPER BACK

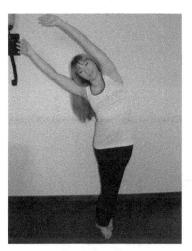

- Stand with your feet together and your posture nice and tall.
- Cross one leg in front of the other.
- Raise your arms high above your head and lean to the side where your foot is crossed.
- Keep your posture nice and tall and pointed forward. Try not to turn your body. Reach as high as you can.

LOW/MID BACK AND SHOULDERS

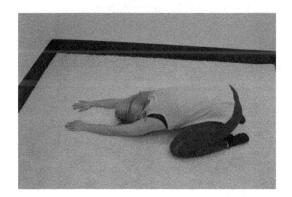

- On your hands and knees, lower your rear end to your heels.
- Reach your hands out above your head and push your chest to the floor.

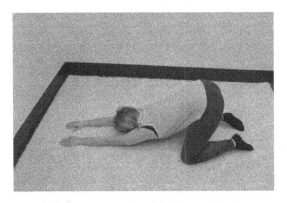

UPPER BACK

- On your hands and knees, slide your hands slightly in front of your head.
- Slowly move your chest down toward the ground keeping your hips up.

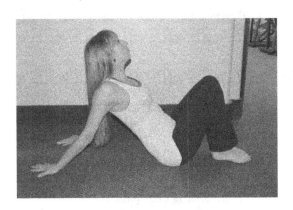

SHOULDERS AND BICEPS

- In a seated position, bend your knees and place your arms behind you.
- Slightly raise your rear end off the ground and slowly move toward your feet until you feel a stretch.
- Lower your rear end to the floor, keeping your back straight. Don't let your chest sink down.

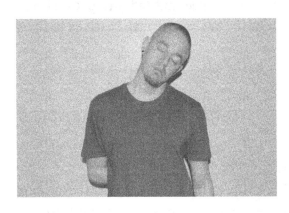

SHOULDER AND NECK

- In a standing or seated position, place your arm behind your back.
- Slowly lean your head to the other side until the stretch is felt.

TENNIS PASSIVE AND STATIC STRETCHING ROUTINE

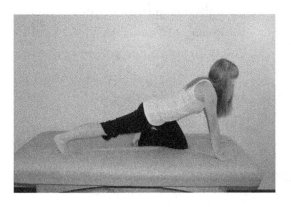

BOTTOM OF FOOT AND CALF

- Start this stretch from your hands and knees.
- Take one leg straight back and place toes on the floor.
- Slowly lean back into your back foot.
- Though you may feel this in your calf as well, ensure that you are focusing on stretching the bottom of the foot.

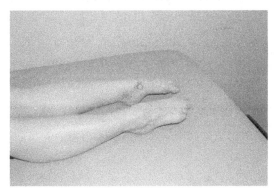 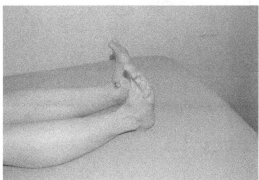

- You can perform this simple dynamic stretch sitting on the floor or in a chair.
- With your legs straight out in front of you, point your toes as far as you can, hold for a second or two, and then pull your toes toward you as far as you can. Repeat 10-15 times.

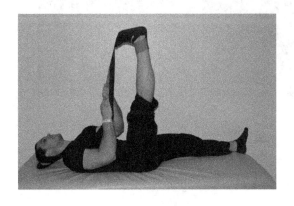

CALF

- Lying flat on your back, place the TStretch strap around your ankle and up the bottom of your foot.
- Bring your leg straight up and pull back and down on the strap.

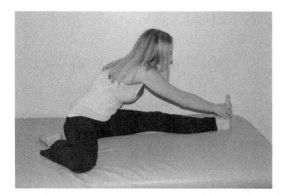

HAMSTRING

- In a seated position, place one leg straight out in front of you. Bend the other leg and place the foot behind you with your knee pointed out.
- Keeping your posture nice and tall, bend forward at the hips.
- Slowly reach for your toes.

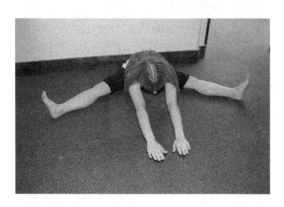

HAMSTRINGS, ADDUCTORS, LOWER BACK

- In a seated position, spread your legs as far as they will go.
- Keeping your posture nice and tall and your toes pointed up, bend forward at the hips.

GLUTES

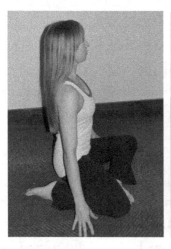 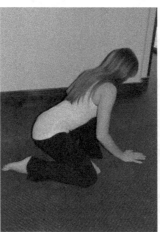 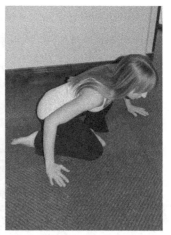

- From a seated position, bend your knee with your foot behind you.
- Bend your opposite leg in front of you and place your foot against the other knee.
- Keeping your posture tall, bend forward at your hips.

HIP FLEXOR, GLUTES, LOWER BACK

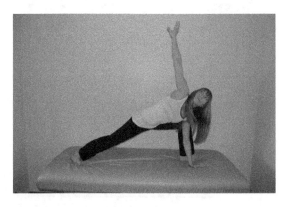

- Place your left leg forward into a lunge position.
- Keeping your right leg straight and your left knee above your heel, lean forward at the hips and place your left hand on the inside of your left foot.
- Pushing your left elbow into your knee, turn your body, and reach to the sky with your right arm.

HIP FLEXOR AND THIGH

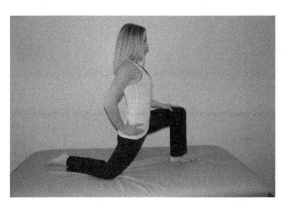

- Get down on both knees and place one foot forward in a lunge position.
- Take your weight down and forward, keeping your posture nice and tall.

HIP AND IT BAND

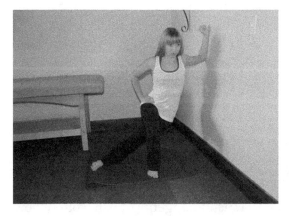

- Stand approximately elbow length away from the wall.
- Take the leg closest to the wall and cross it behind you. Slide it away from the wall as you slowly lower down toward the ground. Do not let your forward knee get past your toes.

UPPER BACK, ABDOMINALS, SHOULDERS

- Hold onto a bar overhead.
- Move your feet backward so your arms are reaching forward.
- Place your weight on your toes and lean forward into the stretch.

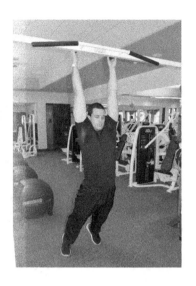

UPPER BACK

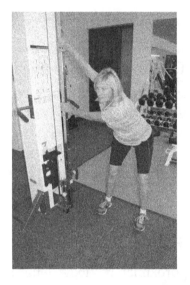

- Begin by standing with your side approximately one foot away from a door jamb or a secure post.
- With your feet shoulder width apart, grasp a door jamb or secure post with both hands (thumbs should point towards each other).
- Place the closest hand on the top about head height and the lower hand even with the lower portion of your chest.
- Making sure your hips are pointed forward, pull with your lower arm, and push with your upper arm.

ROTATOR CUFF

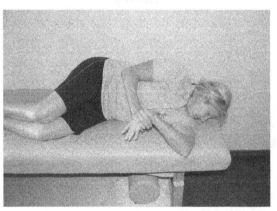

- Lying on your side, bring your arm out to a 90-degree angle. Bend your elbow and wrist also to a 90-degree angle.
- Looking straight down, place your chin on your shoulder.
- Using your other hand, grab your wrist and gently push your elbow down into the ground. Slowly push your hand down toward the floor.

MARTIAL ARTS PASSIVE AND STATIC STRETCHING ROUTINE

CALF

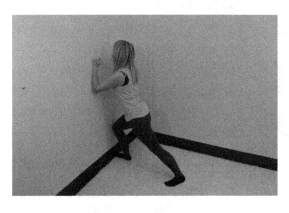

- Begin this stretch by placing the toes of one of your feet at the base of the wall.
- Placing both elbows on the wall, place your other foot a couple of feet behind you with toes pointed forward.
- Slowly lean a bit forward and down, taking your front knee and moving it toward the wall.
- Keep the heel of your back foot on the ground.
- If you can take your front knee to the wall without feeling a stretch, move your back foot back.

HAMSTRING

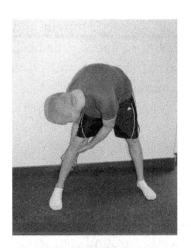

- Stand with your legs straight and a little wider than shoulder-width apart.
- Keeping your posture nice and tall, bend forward at the hips toward the right side.
- Grasp behind the leg and pull down slightly.

ADDUCTOR, GLUTES

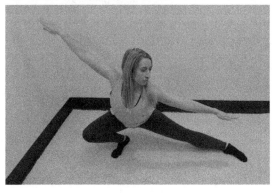

- Spread your legs approximately twice your shoulder width.
- Squat down on the right side, keeping your left leg straight.
- Keeping your arms in a straight line with your left leg, slowly push the inside of your left leg to the ground.

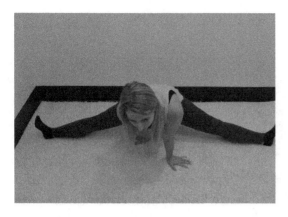

ADDUCTORS

- In a standing position, slowly spread your feet apart.

- Ensuring your toes are pointed up, lower your body as far as you can (into a full split if you are able). Balance yourself by placing your hands on the floor or other stable object.

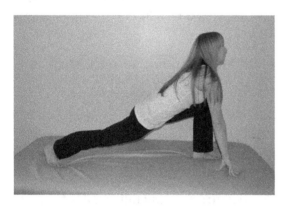

HIP FLEXOR, GLUTES, HAMSTRING

- Standing with your feet together, place one leg forward into a lunge position.

- Keeping your back leg straight and your forward knee above your heel, lean forward at the hips and place both hands on the ground.

- Move your weight down toward the ground.

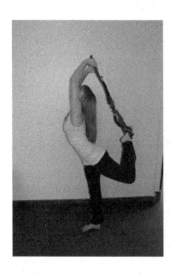

HIP FLEXOR AND THIGH

- Standing with both feet together, bring your foot up behind you and place a strap around your foot.

- Holding onto the strap, bring your hands above your head and pull up and in on your foot.

- With your posture nice and tall and a slight arch in your body, look up toward the ceiling.

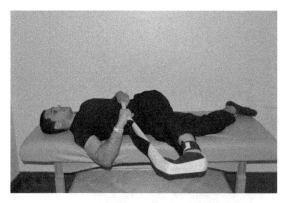

GLUTES AND LOWER BACK

- Place a TStretch strap around your left foot and lie on your right side.
- Holding the strap, keep your left leg straight.
- Slowly push your left shoulder back on the floor/ bed and pull your left leg up toward your head.

GLUTES

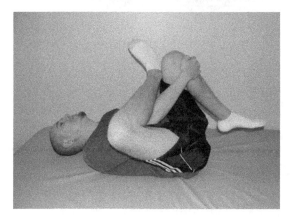

- Lie on your back with both knees bent.
- Place your right ankle on your left knee.
- Take your right arm through your legs and grasp your knee. Take your left hand and place it on your right hand, interlocking your fingers.
- Pull your left knee toward your chest, feeling this stretch in your right hip.

- From a seated position, bend your knee with your foot behind you.
- Bend your opposite leg in front of you and place your foot against the other knee.
- Keeping your posture tall, bend forward at your hips.

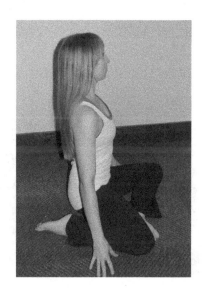

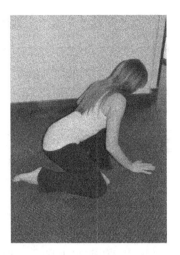 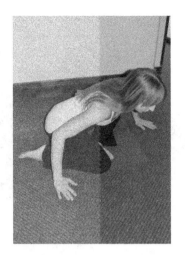

- This is a great stretch because you can lean forward in different directions and stretch different muscles in the hip.

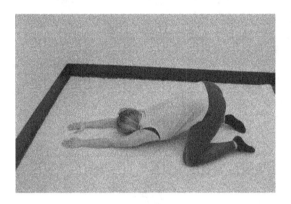

UPPER BACK

- On your hands and knees, slide your hands slightly in front of your head.
- Slowly move your chest down toward the ground keeping your hips up.

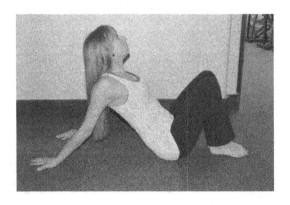

SHOULDERS

- In a seated position, bend your knees and place your arms behind you.
- Slightly raise your rear end off the ground and slowly move toward your feet until you feel a stretch.
- Lower your rear end to the floor, keeping your back straight. Don't let your chest sink down.

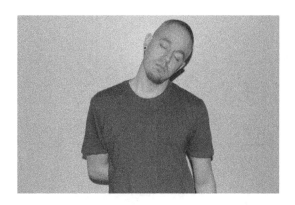

NECK AND SHOULDER

- In a standing or seated position, place your arm behind your back.
- Slowly lean your head to the other side until the stretch is felt.

RECIPES

So what is the point of discussing any kind of nutrition without some recipes? The following recipes were sent to me by celebrity chef Stephanie Izard. Stephanie is best known for being the first female chef to win Bravo's Top Chef. In October of 2011, she published her first cook book, Girl in the Kitchen, and in 2013 she won the James Beard Foundation Award for "Best Chef: Great Lakes". My personal favorite however, was in 2017 when she competed in the first season of Iron Chef Gauntlet. Stephanie won her way up to a spot against Iron Chefs Bobby Flay, Masaharu Morimoto and Michael Simon. She very humbly defeated the three outstanding chefs, earning her the title of Iron Chef. So if you are ever in the Chicago area, please go visit one of her restaurants as she is also Chef/Owner of Girl & The Goat, Little Goat Diner, and Duck Duck Goat.

Herbed Tomato Salad

Yields: 4 servings

- 2 pints Sun Gold cherry tomatoes, halved

- 2 medium/large heirloom tomatoes, cut into 1-inch chunks

- ¼ cup extra-virgin olive oil

- 1 Tbsp fish sauce

- 1 Tbsp red wine vinegar

- ¼ cup roughly chopped mint leaves

- ¼ cup roughly chopped basil leaves

- 2 Tbsp chopped tarragon leaves

- Kosher salt and freshly-cracked black pepper

In a small bowl, whisk together the olive oil, fish sauce, vinegar and a pinch of kosher salt until well combined.

Place tomatoes and herbs in a serving bowl and pour over the vinaigrette. Toss to combine. Season to taste with salt and pepper and serve immediately.

Stephanie loves to serve this with fresh fish!

Pickled Beet Salad

Yields: 4 servings

- 3 cups arugula
- 5 cups baby red oak lettuce, roughly torn
- ½ cup pickled beets (recipe to follow)
- ½ bulb fennel, core removed and thinly sliced (recomended to use a mandoline)
- ½ red onion, thinly sliced (recomended to use a mandoline)
- ½ cup strawberries, sliced
- ¼ cup pepitas (pumpkin needs), toasted
- ¼ cup crumbled goat cheese
- ¼ cup pickling liquid from beets (recipe to follow)
- 2 Tbsp extra-virgin olive oil
- Kosher salt and freshly-cracked black pepper

In a small bowl, whisk together the beet pickling liquid and olive oil. Set aside.

Combine all other ingredients in a large mixing bowl. Pour over the vinegar/oil mixture and toss to combine. Season to taste with salt and pepper and serve immediately.

<u>For Pickled Beets:</u>

- 2 large or 3-4 small golden beets, diced into 1-inch cubes
- 2 garlic cloves, thinly sliced
- 1 cup distilled white vinegar

- ¼ cup granulated sugar

- 1 Tbsp kosher salt

- 1 Tbsp harissa

Place the beets and garlic in a heatproof storage container with a lid.

In a small pot, bring the vinegar and ¼ cup water to a boil over medium heat. Remove from the heat and whisk in the sugar, salt and harissa until the sugar and salt have dissolved. Pour the hot pickling liquid over the beets, making sure they are completely submerged. Let cool at room temperature, then cover and refrigerate overnight, up to 1 month.

Grapefruit Chermoula

Yields: 1 1/2 cups

- 1 cup fresh grapefruit juice

- ¼ cup fresh lime juice

- 2 tsp minced fresh jalapeño

- ¼ cup minced red onion

- 1 tsp minced garlic

- 2 Tbsp chopped fresh cilantro

- 2 Tbsp chopped fresh mint

- ½ tsp kosher salt, plus more to taste

Place all ingredients in a mixing bowl and toss to combine. Season to taste with salt.

Stephanie loves to serve this drizzled over fresh avocados, alongside fish or meat!

Sautéed Eggplant

Yields: 4 servings

- 3-4 Japanese eggplants

- 2 Tbsp balsamic vinegar

- 2 Tbsp soy sauce or Tamari

- 1 Tbsp Shaoxing rice wine

- 1 tsp Asian chili paste, such as Sambal Oelek

- ¼ cup canola or rice bran oil

- Pickled Frenos chilis (recipe to follow), for topping

- Toasted sesame seeds, for topping

- Fresh mint leaves, for topping

Trim the tops and bottoms off of the eggplant. Cut into quarters, lengthwise, then cut crosswise into 2-inch pieces.

In a small mixing bowl, whisk together the vinegar, Shaoxing, soy sauce and Sambal.

Heat a large sauté pan or wok over medium-high heat and add in the oil. Once the oil is hot (but not smoking), add in the eggplant in a single layer (working in batches if necessary), tossing to coat in the oil. Season with a pinch of kosher salt. Continue sautéing, flipping occasionally, until the eggplant is well browned on all sides and tender.

Once most of the oil has been absorbed, deglaze the pan with the vinaigrette mixture. Continue cooking, tossing eggplant around in the sauce, until well-glazed and most of the liquid has been absorbed.

Transfer to a serving plate. Top with pickled Fresnos, toasted sesame seeds and fresh mint leaves. Serve warm or at room temperature.

For Pickled Fresnos:

- 1 cup sliced and seeded Fresno chiles

- ⅔ cup champagne vinegar

- ¼ cup sugar

- 1 tsp kosher salt

Place Fresnos in a heat-proof storage container with a lid. Add the vinegar, sugar and salt to a medium saucepan and bring to a boil over medium-high heat. Pour the hot liquid over the fresnos, making sure they are completely submerged. Let cool completely at room temperature, then cover and refrigerate until ready to serve.

Grilled Corn on the Cob

Yields: 4 servings

- 4 ears of corn, shucked and cleaned
- ¼ cup (4 Tbsp) unsalted butter, softened
- 1 tsp cayenne pepper
- Kosher salt
- ¼ cup grated Parmesan cheese
- 2 limes, halved
- ¼ cup cilantro leaves, roughly chopped

First, make your compound butter by mixing the cayenne pepper and a pinch of kosher salt into the softened butter until well combined.

Preheat a grill or grill-pan to medium-high heat. Place corn on the grill (no need to toss it in any oil first, it will get plenty of butter later). Let cook, rotating frequently, until the kernels turn bright yellow and begin to likely char on each side, about 1-2 minutes per side.

Remove corn and place lime halves on the grill, cut-side down. Grill until warmed through and light char marks appear, about 2 minutes.

Meanwhile, while the corn is still hot, brush liberally with cayenne-spiced compound butter.

Sprinkle with Parmesan cheese and freshly-chopped cilantro. Squeeze warm lime juice over the top and dig in!

CONCLUSION

If you have ever read any articles or books written by Harvey Mackay, you know he is full of wisdom and wit. At the end of his articles and sections in his books, he always provides great one liners and wonderful advice which is entitled "Mackay's Moral." If you have never read him before, I would highly suggest you do ... he is great. In his book *You Haven't Hit Your Peak Yet*, he provides you with some original thoughts, two of which fit this book to a T!

The most crippling disease: Excuses.
The greatest natural resource: Our youth.

I do not want to preach to you, but isn't this true? We have all become so busy that we create so many excuses for why we cannot do things, even if we know it is good for us. You, however, have taken a step to better yourself by purchasing this book. Now you must get to work and carve out some time at least 10-20 minutes, 4-5 days a week to dedicate to your stretching – No Excuses. I assure you that if you can accomplish this, you cannot help but feel more invigorated in every step, side shuffle, swing, and jump. You never know, you may even be like my client I mentioned earlier and even feel more youthful again.

This book is meant to give you a jump start into your new stretching program as well as provide you with some basic knowledge of how and why stretching works. I hope you use this book as your resource for new stretches and stretching programs. I would also encourage you to purchase the T-Stretch strap and get familiar with it. Not only will it allow you to stretch muscles in a totally different way, taking stress off your body, but it will also assist you in stretching muscles that are difficult to stretch any other way.

I would also encourage you to leave this book, strap, and a foam roller out in the open so you can see it every day and use it as a reminder for what you need to get done. You know what they say, "out of sight, out of mind"! I wish you the best of luck, I know you can do it. Follow along with your program, remember to hold each stretch for 20-30 seconds and don't forget to breathe.

ABOUT THE AUTHOR

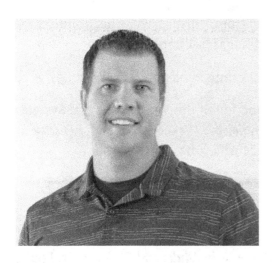

Aaron Taylor is a flexibility therapist with 20 years of experience. Within this time, he has developed a keen eye and feel for the human body. After working with individuals with knee replacements and hip replacements to individuals afflicted with Parkinson's Disease and Polio, Aaron has seen it all.

His clients have ranged from 12-year-old kids and 93-year-old weekend warriors to individuals with motor muscular deficiencies and joint replacements. Aaron has also developed a long list of some of the biggest names in the business world as well as sport and entertainment history. He has been featured in American Fitness Magazine and has also appeared in Sports Illustrated alongside Muhammad Ali.

In addition, Aaron has designed the TStretch strap that is used to assist individuals with their everyday stretching program.

Born and raised in Alamosa, Colorado, Aaron played sports from his earliest years; football, basketball, wrestling, and baseball - but the discovery of golf at the age of six became Aaron's passion. Playing throughout high school, he went on to become a three time All-Conference golfer for Adams State University where he received his Bachelor's degree in Sport and Exercise Management. During his Master's program in Health, Aaron coached the Adams State golf team, helping them achieve their first ever top 10 ranking.

BIBLIOGRAPHY

18 Foods and Drinks That Are Surprisingly High In Sugar. *Healthline.* 2016 July 18; [cited 2016 Nov 18] Available from: https://www.healthline.com/nutrition/18-surprising-foods-high-in-sugar#section2.

Braverman, R. Eric. *The Edge Effect.* New York: Sterling Publishing Co Inc; 2005. 195 p.

Crowther – Radulewicz CL. Structure and Function of the Musculoskeletal System. In: McCance KL, Huether SE. *Pathophysiology: The Biologic Basis for Disease in Adults and Children.* St. Lous: El Sevier Mosby; 2014. p. 1520, 1536.

Coulter, H. David. Anatomy of Hatha Yoga. Marlboro: Body & Breath Inc. 2001

Cunningham SG, Brashers VL, McCance KL. Structure and Function of the Cardiovascular and Lymphatic System. In: McCance KL, Huether SE. *Pathophysiology: The Biologic Basis for Disease in Adults and Children.* St. Louis: El Sevier Mosby; 2014. p. 1108.

Heslin, Jo-Ann., & Natow, Annette. The Most Complete Food Counter: 2nd Edition. New York: Simon & Schuster, 2011.

Holick, F. Michael. Sunlight and Vitamin D: Both Good for Cardiovascular Health. *Journal of General Internal Medicine.* 2002 Sep; 17(9): 733-735

Lombardo, Gerard. *Sleep To Save Your Life: The Complete Guide to Living Longer and Healthier Through Restorative Sleep.* New York: Harper Collins; 2005. p. 22-23, 91.

My Food Data: Be Healthy. *My Food Data.* 2019; [cited 2019 June 28] Available from: https://www.myfooddata.com.

Nolan KJ, Heslin JA. The Complete Food Counter 4th ed. New York: Simon & Schuster Inc; 2012. 26 p.

Shutterstock, Inc. Web site [Internet]. New York (NY): Shutterstock; [cited 2020 May 16]. Available from: https://www.shutterstock.com.

This Just In: Over Consumption of Sugar Contributes to Muscle and Joint Pain. *Virginia Therapy & Fitness Center* 2015 Nov 6; [cited 2017 June 29] Available from: http://www.spinemd.com/vtfc/news/this-just-in-over-consumption-of-sugar-contributes-to-muscle-joint-pain.

Understanding The Importance of Proper Hydration For Maximum Gains In And Out Of The Gym. *Bodybuilding.* 2019; [cited 2019 July 24] Available from: https://www.bodybuilding.com/fun/behar12.htm.

Vitamin C. *Merck Manual Professional Version.* 2018 March; [cited 2018 May 7]. Available from: https;//www.merckmanuals.com/professional/nutritional-disorders/vitamin-deficiency,-dependecy,-and-toxicity/vitamin-c.

END NOTES

1. Cunningham, 1108
2. p. 1536
3. Crowther p.1520
4. Holick, p. 2-3
5. Merck Manual
6. Nolan
7. Braverman (2004)
8. Article "18 Foods and Drinks That Are Surprisingly High In Sugar" (Need Magazine or book citation)
9. Lombardo, 2005

CPSIA information can be obtained
at www.ICGtesting.com
Printed in the USA
BVHW010227120122
626062BV00010B/353